SPECIAL TREATMENT

How to Get the
Same High-Quality Health Care
Your Doctor Gets

SPECIAL TREATMENT

How to Get the
Same High-Quality Health Care
Your Doctor Gets

KEVIN J. SODEN, M.D., M.P.H.,
and CHRISTINE DUMAS, D.D.S.

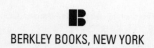
BERKLEY BOOKS, NEW YORK

B

A Berkley Book
Published by The Berkley Publishing Group
A division of Penguin Group (USA) Inc.
375 Hudson Street
New York, New York 10014

Copyright © 2003 by Dr. Kevin J. Soden and Dr. Christine Dumas
Cover design by Richard Hasselberger
Cover photograph © 2003 by Jan Cobb
Book design by Tiffany Estreicher

PRINTING HISTORY
Berkley hardcover edition: September 2003
Berkley trade paperback edition: September 2004
Berkley trade paperback ISBN: 0-425-19809-X

The Library of Congress has catalogued the Berkley hardcover edition as follows:

Soden, Kevin.
    Special treatment: ten ways to get the same high-quality health care your doctor gets / Kevin J. Soden and Christine Dumas.
    p. cm
    Includes index.
    ISBN 0-425-19168-0
    1. Medical care—Miscellanea. I. Dumas, Christine. II. Title.
RA395 .A3 S724 2003   2003056019
395—dc21

PRINTED IN THE UNITED STATES OF AMERICA
10 9 8 7 6 5 4 3 2 1

CONTENTS

INTRODUCTION

Do you ever wish you had a doctor in the family? Someone you could call when you have a health emergency; someone to be your advocate when you go for surgery; someone to ask the right questions during a doctor's visit; or someone to tell you the very best specialist to go to in case of a serious problem? We bet you do. After a total of forty years in our respective fields, we don't know anyone whose life hasn't been touched by some illness or medical problem, whether it be a family member or personally.

We think you'd like to have a doctor in your family because doctors have a built-in advantage when it comes to navigating the health care system. This is especially true in this era of managed care and all its accompanying frustrations. When a doctor goes to see another doctor, or when a doctor goes into the hospital, the process, treatment, and information exchanged are, quite simply, very different than what happens to your average patient. Doctors and their families get extra-special care that the rest of us just don't have access to. When they get sick, or have a medical emergency, or just need to maintain their own health or that of their families, their knowledge and connections help them to get better faster and sooner than almost anyone else.

There's a mystique attached to medicine that both awes and confuses most people not on the inside. It's the same way the average person feels about television and the movies. Who doesn't want to be able to look behind the cameras and see how it's done and what's behind the scenes? Sometimes by learning how things are really done and how they really work, the magic fades. We learn that the reality of how TV shows or movies are made has little resemblance to what we finally see on our TV sets or on the silver screen. This can be both good and bad. It can take away our innocence, but in the process, it can help us to be more appreciative of the skills that the performers and filmmakers possess. In the end, we become better consumers and our standards and expectations are raised.

Similarly, have you ever wanted to "pull back the curtain" on medicine, peek behind the scenes, and get an insider's look? Well, that is what this book is all about. We know that doctors and their families often get treated differently than the average patient or consumer of health care. Why? It's because they know things that we don't know. They know what really happens on the "inside."

Getting an "insider's" view of medicine is more difficult than for most other professions. There are several reasons for our inability to crack the secret code of medicine. First, medical information is very personal and is treated with strict confidentiality. People want to protect the privacy of their health care information, and the profession has done an excellent job of maintaining that secrecy. Second, the language and the knowledge base needed to understand what is happening is formidable, and this has kept most people uninformed. The long, complicated, scientific terms used in medicine add to the confusion of the average person. No one wants to appear stupid, so they don't ask questions and, until recently, relied totally on their doctors. Third, the medical profession has done a very good job of taking care of people and putting the patient first. As a result, most patients haven't worried too much about whose interest the doctor is putting first. Now, thanks to the competing interests of managed care organizations—the patient and the bottom-line cost—doctors are often caught in the middle. This has eroded some of the traditional trust patients have in the medical profession. You can't serve two masters all the time.

With *Special Treatment,* we want to demystify the medical profession and help you to appreciate the magic of medicine even more. We want you to learn what doctors know that the average patient doesn't know. We want to help you peek behind the curtains and see what most people don't get to experience. We're going to use our over forty years of medical experience in both clinical practice and medical reporting to provide you the kind of "inside" information you need.

Why is this so important for you? It's very simple. We all will either be a patient ourselves or will have a family member who requires medical care. We all will have to participate in the system. We all will be affected at some point in time by our experiences with the health care system. (Let us, your authors, assure you that we both have had some very positive and negative experiences with health care, so trust us, we can relate to what we are writing.)

Why are we qualified to write this book and how do we know this kind of inside information? Christine is a dentist who's been doing health-related stories on television for twelve years. Kevin is a physician who spent twenty-five years in an emergency room and has been a medical reporter for eighteen years. As national health care reporters for NBC News, we've had the opportunity to interview some of the best and the brightest physicians and health care professionals that the finest medical system in the world has to offer. We want to share the secrets we have learned in our own practices, the information we have gleaned from our interviews, the knowledge we've gained from working within the health care system, and the important, very personal lessons that we've learned from our fellow doctors and patients. In other words, we want this book to be like having a doctor in your very own family.

In this book, we will provide you with information that doctors know . . . and that most other people don't. Some of this information may surprise you. Your doctor might not know some of this information either.

It's not a knock on him or her, but may simply be something they've never thought about since they're on the inside already.

We'll give you an inside look at hospitals, emergency rooms, surgery, and how your doctor makes a diagnosis. We'll also focus on the medical problems that kill almost 80 percent of Americans and will affect most of us at some time in our lives. We intend to provide you with some information that you can use right now. We'll also give you the information you'll need to do some more research on your own and to get the answers you need in order to have a positive impact on your health. It's medical news that you can use.

Some of what we'll say and what you'll learn in this book will be controversial. We know that some people or some groups won't like our honesty and the way we see things, so they'll take potshots at us. We don't care. What we want to do is help you. We've been given the gift and the privilege of caring for people. Our patients have trusted us with their lives and with the intimate aspects of their lives. We owe you the same knowledge that we have and hope that it has a positive impact on your health.

We know that this book will make you think, and we hope that it helps you begin a dialogue with your health care provider. Ultimately, what you decide and how you act about your medical care may be different from what we may suggest, but now you're going to be making that decision with more knowledge and with an "insider's" look at medicine. So, let's lift the curtain and enter the secret world of medicine together.

CHAPTER ONE

Choosing A Primary Care Doctor and Getting the Best Specialist Care

Dr. Justice arrived at the emergency room shortly after his patient did. The ER staff wasn't surprised, as Dr. Justice and his medical colleagues always liked to care for their own patients when possible. The patient had called Dr. Justice (who had returned his phone call promptly) to tell him that he had chest pain. Dr. Justice told him to call 911 and get to the ER by ambulance. He would call the ER, give them some orders, and would follow along shortly.

Dr. Justice spoke with his patient in a calm and unhurried manner and assured him that he would get the best possible medical care. He and his medical group would oversee each step of his care in consultation with the specialists in the hospital—the same specialists that he would use if it were for himself.

Dr. Justice then invited the patient's wife into the examining room with her husband and reassured her in the same quiet, confident manner as he had reassured her husband. He held her hand while sitting in the chair next to her, all the while listening to her *concerns. He addressed each question in a respectful and easy style that immediately calmed the worried wife. Finally, when she had all her questions answered, he hugged her and left the room to see another patient. The nursing staff could see an immediate positive difference in the whole family after Dr. Justice had finished.*

Who wouldn't want a doctor like this? Sound like a fantasy doctor from Central Casting? Well, it's not. There are many wonderful doctors in the practice of medicine who provide this same kind of caring and compassion. This is the kind of care we'd all like to have and deserve to have. It is possible to find a doctor or doctors like the one in our little scenario. It will take some time and effort on your part, but it's possible.

THINK ABOUT THIS:
- The number of physicians in the United States is 700,000.
- The number of accidental deaths caused by physicians per year is 120,000.
- The number of accidental deaths per physician is 0.171 per year.

(Health and Human Services Dept.)

THEN THINK ABOUT THIS:
- The number of gun owners in the United States is 80 million.
- The number of accidental gun deaths per year (all age groups) is 1,500.
- The number of accidental deaths per gun owner per year is .0000188.

Statistically, doctors are approximately nine thousand times more dangerous than gun owners. FACT: Not everyone has a gun, but almost everyone has at least one doctor.

The above is a joke making its way around the Internet that might just contain a bit of truth. It's a humorous way of letting you know that finding the right doctor is extremely important to your health because, according to a 1998 Gallup Poll, 83 percent of Americans visited a doctor in the previous year. While most people saw a doctor for routine care of common problems, many others required a specialist's care for more serious and complex issues.

The biggest problem that many people have in medical care is finding the right doctor. In survey after survey, people have defined the "right" doctor as one who is compassionate, kind, listens to what they are saying, and includes them as partners in their treatment. Many of us are blessed with a doctor we can trust and who provides wonderful care for us and our families. Many others of us are not.

We won't kid you. Finding the right doctor for you can be hard work. It takes time and may require considerable effort. In some cases, you may get lucky and strike gold right away. It's good to keep in mind that anything good and worth having in life usually requires some work, and the feeling of accomplishment you get when the job is done and you find the right doctor makes it all worthwhile. After all, in this case, we're talking about your health and maybe your life.

BUYING A CAR AND FINDING A DOCTOR

How many of you have bought a car in the last several years? We bet most of you have. Did you do a fair amount of research before you bought your car? We bet you did, because a car is something you live with for years, and it's one of the biggest dollar outlays that a person makes other than the purchase of their home.

When you finished doing your research by talking to friends, looking at car ratings on the Internet, in *Consumer Reports,* or whatever other rating service you decided to use, did you then take your finalists out for a test drive? We bet you did that too, because by doing so, you noticed little things about the car that you couldn't have found out by simply reading or talking to someone else about it. It doesn't matter that someone else loves a particular car model; your car has to fit your personality and be comfortable for you.

Those who sell cars and trucks know that the average consumer also makes their final decision about the vehicle they choose based on a number of intangibles. Was the sales staff nice? Did one dealer promise better service after the sale than another? Was the dealer's showroom clean and appealing? Is the dealership convenient? Does the dealer have a reputation in town for honesty and caring service? Did the particular car and model have a reputation for reliability and good service?

Let's take that same analogy and apply it to choosing a doctor. How much time and effort did you take before choosing your present doctor or a doctor that you've seen in the past? Did you do your research by checking out your doctor through the state medical society, specialty board, or on the Internet? If not, why not? You may not make a big dollar investment in your doctor, thanks to insurance, but aren't you potentially investing your life (and possibly your family's lives) in your doctor's hands? We think you are, and that's why we think this chapter is so important.

Did you take the doctors you are considering out for a test drive by scheduling a brief meeting with them in their offices? You may find that despite all your research, the doctor's support staff or office left a lot to be desired. You may find that the office hours just weren't convenient and that your potential future doctor wasn't available after standard office hours or didn't have coverage in emergencies. Maybe, when you sat in the waiting room prior to your appointment, some of the other patients mentioned some concerns they had about the care they'd received. These are some of the things that you can find out only when visiting your potential doctor's office personally. Isn't it worth your time to do so? You do it when you're buying a car. Why not when choosing the person who will have an even greater impact on your life?

How do you find the best doctor for you? When do you need a second opinion? When should you consult a specialist for care? What kinds of questions should you ask when looking for a doctor? These questions, and more, are at the heart of this most important chapter.

FINDING THE BEST DOCTOR AND GETTING THE KIND OF CARE YOUR DOCTOR GETS

Getting the best care isn't really just a function of how much money you have. What you need is something more important . . . information. And the very best kind of information when it comes to health care is insider information. The good news here is that in the world of medicine insider information is legal . . . and that's what we want to share with you.

So who has this insider information? Doctors do. Doctors definitely have the inside track when it comes to finding the best doctors and getting the best care. Your friends who are doctors know who the best doctors are, how to get in to see them quickly and without waiting, and how to get referrals to the best specialists, if and when they need them.

The key to staying healthy and out of the hospital is to be in the hands of the best primary care physician you can find. Most of us have no idea how to find one or how to evaluate one once we join their practice. Doctors, on the other hand, spend their lives in clinical settings. They know their way around the world of health care the way a professional golfer knows his way around a golf course.

Very simply, the way most people go about choosing a doctor is all wrong. And it is one of the costliest errors that you can make. There isn't anything more important to most of us than our health and the health of the people we love. When we are diagnosed with an illness or even when we're choosing a physician to take care of us, we want nothing less than the best, and the best care starts with your primary care physician.

YOUR PRIMARY CARE PHYSICIAN: THE MOST IMPORTANT MEMBER OF YOUR HEALTH CARE TEAM

Your primary care physician is the most important person on your health care team. This doctor will be the coordinator of your overall medical care much like a head chef oversees the kitchen staff in fine restaurants or an executive producer manages and coordinates the *Today* show every day.

When the *Today* show airs, there is an executive producer who coordinates all the various story segments and program features and brings them together into a final product that flows seamlessly. He or she might be coordinating twenty or more features with as many different producers. This is a very difficult job because it means limiting certain stories and expanding others in the hope of appealing to the widest possible audience five days a week, fifty-two weeks a year. We wouldn't want that job. It's just too stressful.

Your primary doctor provides much the same role for you. He or she should be supervising all aspects of your medical care and ensuring that all members of the team blend together to provide the best health care for you. It too is a very difficult and stressful job because other team members may not communicate with the primary care provider as they should, reports may get lost, and results may be slow in getting back to the doctor's office. And, if things should go wrong, the primary physician is often second-guessed, especially with the twenty-twenty hindsight that many people develop. A doctor who does this job well is to be respected and cherished.

Your primary care provider should be your initial contact for almost all your medical problems and will be responsible for evaluating, diagnosing, and treating your various illnesses and ailments. If necessary, they are often responsible for referring you to a specialist for more advanced care. Many managed care organizations (MCOs) call this latter role being a "gatekeeper." If you don't get the approval of your primary doctor before going to

Useful Terms to Know

Board Certified: Doctors who are board certified have had specialized training and have gone through a rigorous evaluation process, including an examination designed to demonstrate a certain level of knowledge in a certain field of medicine. This includes family practice, pediatrics, OB-GYN, surgery, internal medicine, and geriatrics, to mention several of the main groups. There are thirty-six areas of medicine that are certified by the American Board of Medical Specialties. For more information about this process and the specialties go to www.abms.org/approved.asp.

Board Eligible: Doctors can call themselves board eligible in a particular field if they have been trained in a certain specialty but have not taken (or have not passed) the examination for that specialty.

Licensed: A physician must be licensed in each state where he or she practices medicine. You can be licensed in more than one state at the same time. If a physician is not licensed in a state, he is legally not allowed to practice in that state. State boards of medical examiners are the only groups who can license a physician.

Recertification in a Medical Specialty: All specialty certifications issued today are limited to between six to ten years. This means that a doctor must recertify or pass another examination to maintain his specialty status. If he does not do so, he can still practice medicine but cannot call himself a board-certified specialist. Trust us on this point . . . you always want to be cared for by a doctor who is board certified and has maintained that certification.

a specialist, then the MCO will pay substantially less (or not at all) for that care. By placing the primary care physician in the "gatekeeper" role, the MCOs often avoid unnecessary and costly specialist care because a good primary care doctor can handle most medical problems that you have.

HOW TO GO ABOUT SELECTING YOUR PRIMARY CARE PHYSICIAN

Let's take a minute and look at an event that happens to millions of Americans each month. You're moving. It can be to another city or to the other side of town. It doesn't matter. One way or another, you are being uprooted. You are going from the familiar to something new and different. There are many adjustments that have to take place—some good and some not so good—and all these changes can be potentially stressful.

One of the biggest concerns that we hear from people when they move from one place to another is "How am I going to find another doctor that's as wonderful as the one I have now? I don't know anyone in this new city, so how will I know who's good and who's not good?" We know this is traumatic, but we also know that we can help make the job of finding a new doctor less stressful for you.

If you've got children, if you've got some chronic medical problems, or if you're just concerned about taking good care of yourself, when you move, you need to find another doctor immediately. How do you go about it? First of all, let us say, there is no quick or easy way to go about this if you want to do the job right. Sure, you could go to the list of doctors that most companies provide through their health benefit plan and blindly pick a name off the list. Needless to say, we don't suggest that approach. We think there is a better way to find the best doctor for you.

Before you go about doing anything, you need to decide what kind of doctor you really want. What are your preferences? Do you want a male or female physician? Do you want a group practice or a solo practice? Do you want someone older or younger? Do you want someone who practices in a particular hospital? Most of us have preferences about the kind of person we want caring for us. You need to define them or else any doctor will do (and we know that's not the case). So, let's get started and let's find the right doctor for you.

First, if you have a doctor in your previous location, ask him or her if they know a good doctor in the new city. They may not, but sometimes they do, and that can shorten your search. Either way, it's worth a try, and you just might get lucky. Even if she doesn't know a primary care specialist, there may be another doctor in the city whom she knows and trusts and who can give you the names of some doctors.

Second, when you get to your new location, ask your neighbors what doctor they use and how they feel about him or her. You can learn a lot from their experiences. If you're at a new job, new church, or school, ask your coworkers, church members, or parents in the school if they have any preferences for doctors. Get them to explain what they like and don't like about their choices. You can often get some great leads this way.

Third, most hospitals have referral lists of available physicians that they will provide to you. When you speak to someone from the hospital, ask that person where he or she goes for medical care. Hospital personnel often know the good doctors from the bad. Don't hesitate to ask why they like the doctor they recommend.

You also have some choices to make about the type of primary care specialist that will care for you. Do you want a family practice physician (a doctor who cares for all family members regardless of age), an internist (a doctor trained in general medicine who cares only for adults), or a geriatrician (a physician trained to care for older adults). It really doesn't matter which of these doctors you choose as long as they are board certified and are skilled in caring for your particular medical problems.

After gathering some names, look these doctors up on the Internet and begin doing some research on them. Are they licensed in your state? Are they board certified? Do they have any disciplinary actions against them from the state board of medical examiners? Did they attend a reputable medical school? Have they published any papers in medical journals?

Here are some Web sites that can be useful in helping you evaluate your doctor.

www.docboard.org: This site is run by a consortium of thirty state medical boards and provides some very helpful public information about particular doctors. The quality of the data varies from state to state and is largely based on public documents. For instance, the Massachusetts site provides information reported by the doctors themselves. It is not checked for accuracy, so the data can potentially be old or incomplete, and not tell the whole story. The North Carolina board site provides data found only in public documents, while the Maryland site provides more extensive data about doctors.

www.abms.org: The American Board of Medical Specialties provides information on this site. It is a good, free site that tells you whether or not a physician is board certified and what that means. When a doctor is board certified, it means that he has demonstrated a certain basic level of competency in his particular specialty. Some specialties like family practice and emergency medicine require recertification every several years, while others require no recertification or proof of competency (hard to believe, isn't it?).

www.fsmb.org: The Federation of State Medical Boards is a consortium of all state medical boards.

Fourth, phone the office of all the doctors you are considering and ask some basic questions. Is the doctor accepting new patients? Will another doctor be available to treat you when your doctor is off? What happens in emergency situations? What are the office hours? What insurance does she take?

Last (and we think the most important step), make an appointment to meet and interview the doctor. We know this may take considerable time and effort (and possibly some money), but this is the most important step in finding a doctor you can trust and care for you.

Think back to when you were dating. You often knew within a few minutes whether or not you wanted to see someone again. By being in their presence and seeing how they interacted with you, you immediately knew on both a conscious and unconscious level whether you clicked with that person. The same thing occurs when you meet your doctor. Here are a few questions you need to ask yourself when meeting with a potential doctor:

- Does the doctor really listen to what I'm trying to say or does he or she interrupt before my thoughts are finished?

- Do I feel rushed by the doctor?

- Are his/her thoughts about wellness or prevention similar to mine?

- Do I feel comfortable in his/her presence?

- Was I treated courteously and with respect?

- Were my questions answered honestly and without being evaded?

As we mentioned above, there are some other things to consider when selecting a PCP, such as the location of the doctor's office (Is it convenient?); the hospital where a doctor admits his or her patients (Is it the best hospital for your care?); the health plans he or she takes (Do you have to pay more by going to this doctor?); the age, race, and sex of your doctor; his or her understanding of your cultural background; and the languages that the doctor speaks. You have to decide what factors are most important to you and make your final selection based on them.

Trust your gut instincts when reviewing your visit with the doctor. They are more often right than not. And, don't make a final selection about a doctor until you interview a few physicians. Your health is just too important to be left to chance.

WHEN IS IT TIME TO LOOK FOR ANOTHER DOCTOR OR SPECIALIST?

In the course of interviewing patients and speaking to friends, we often hear horror stories about medical care gone awry or doctor-patient relationships that are less than optimal. All relationships can't be perfect, and dealing with a doctor is no different. Sometimes you need to find another doctor because things just aren't working with the one you've got or you need help from a specialist. What are some of the signs and symptoms of a doctor-patient relationship in trouble or needing assistance?

Communication between you and your doctor is mediocre at best: Getting the best medical care requires high-level communication between both parties that is characterized by trust, careful listening to the other, and respect. If these traits are absent or sorely lacking, it's time to move on, provided the problem lies with your doctor. If the problems in communication are your fault, then finding another doctor won't make any difference.

The information you receive from your doctor is inaccurate: No doctor can be perfect because there is just too much information for one person to know. What you can expect is that your doctor is right almost all the time or he or she tells you, "I don't know but I will find out, or I can direct you to someone who does know." If you don't trust your doctor's opinion, then you need to go elsewhere.

Your doctor lies or is evasive: You should expect honesty and directness from your health care provider. If either of these is lacking after you've confronted your doctor about them, then find someone else.

You're not making progress with a particular medical problem: Sometimes looking at a problem with a new set of eyes and ears is all it takes to get to find a solution. We're sure you've seen this in many situations.

You're struggling with a problem and then someone walks in and almost immediately comes up with a solution. It's not that they're smarter than you, it's just that they can view the problem from a different perspective. And if your doctor is having trouble treating you, it doesn't mean that she is incompetent. Ask to be referred to a specialist for a second opinion. This won't threaten good doctors if what they're doing isn't working. They know everyone needs help at times. Doctors also know that asking for a specialist's opinion is one of the best ways to learn.

Your doctor never has time to answer your questions adequately: Wherever we go today, it seems like everyone is in a rush. Managed care organizations want doctors to see more patients in less time so they can make more money. Doctors sometimes have as little as eight minutes per patient to evaluate, diagnose, and treat a person. It doesn't leave much time for questions. Despite this, good doctors make the time to address your concerns. If your doctor doesn't have time for you, you don't have time for him or her either.

Keep these warning signs in mind and take action if you notice them in your relationship with your doctor. When you are ready to discharge your doctor and go to another, you should formally ask in writing that your records be transferred to another doctor's office. If you don't have another doctor yet, ask that a copy of all your records be available for you. If the doctor's office doesn't want to give you a copy, then have them mailed to another doctor when you finally select one. We also suggest that you indicate the reasons why you are leaving in your letter in hopes that your doctor will address your concerns; if not with you, he or she might change their behavior in the future, if appropriate. Only about 25 percent of patients ever tell their doctors why they are leaving the practice. If more patients explained why they were displeased, there is a better chance that a doctor would make some changes.

What we all want is a mutual relationship built on respect and trust with a caring, compassionate doctor. Part of the reason we don't get some of what we need from some doctors is because they don't learn it in medical school. One of the things that patients often assume is that because their doctor has gone to medical school and has M.D. after his name, he's learned a great deal about all aspects of medicine. This couldn't be further from the truth. Medical schools are so focused on the science aspects of medicine that students learn little, if anything, about many of the subjects that patients are extremely concerned about.

Why are we telling you all this? We want you to realize that there is no way that any doctor can be all things to all patients, so don't develop unrealistic expectations. Instead, make sure to ask your doctor his or her views on the following areas:

- The art of medicine: learning how to care for and listen to patients

- Death and dying: treating those dying to improve their quality of life

- Spirituality

- Physical therapy and rehabilitation: maximizing a person's return to normal functioning after a medical illness or surgery

- Obesity care

- Nutrition, diets, and herbal supplements

- Alternative medicines: what we can learn from nontraditional approaches to a problem

It's not a knock on your doctor if she is not proficient in some or all of these areas. It simply means that if you need this kind of help, you need to ask for a referral to someone more skilled in this area.

WOMEN: ARE THEY BEING SHORTCHANGED WHEN IT COMES TO PRIMARY CARE?

What we're going to say here will be controversial and we know it. Women are often shortchanged when it comes to the kind of primary medical care they receive. We know what most of you are thinking: "They can't be serious. They just don't know what they're talking about." Well, we are serious and we do know what we're talking about . . . and what we do know is that many women are not getting the total medical care that they deserve. We hope we've got your attention now.

A great many women operate under the assumption that if they see their OB-GYN doctors (mainly their gynecologist) every year, they are getting all the medical care they need. That is just not the case. A gynecologist is great if you're only interested in female problems or just what happens below your waist. The problem is that the number one killer of women is cardiovascular disease, and most OB-GYN doctors don't have the time in a routine ob-gyn visit to diagnose and treat cardiovascular disease and the risk factors associated with it. (See Chapter 8 to learn more.)

We strongly believe that if women choose to see their OB-GYN for care of many female-related problems, then they definitely must have a second physician, such as a family practice specialist or an internal medicine specialist, provide the rest of their care. If not, too many problems may be overlooked or not addressed proactively.

The bottom line: We don't care where women get their care. We just want to make sure they get all their health care issues addressed. Right now too many

> The best doctors know that surgery should be a last option and utilized only after all other options have been exhausted

women are being shortchanged in their medical care and that's what we'd like to see changed.

CHOOSING THE RIGHT DOCTOR FOR YOUR CHILD

Children are not just little adults. Children's medical needs and issues are definitely different. Like adults, children do have different problems and needs based upon a particular stage in their life. Babies are different from children, who are different from teens. Pediatricians and family practice specialists deliver the majority of care to children of all ages. So, what should a parent do to pick a doctor for their child? Outside of evaluating the basic medical skills of the doctor you are considering, there are some other questions you should consider asking. We advise doing the same thing you do when picking a doctor for yourself: conduct an interview with your child's potential doctor.

The environment of any doctor's office can provide huge insights into whether or not you want that doctor caring for your child. Are there separate waiting rooms to keep sick children away from well children or adults? Is the waiting room clean and kid friendly? Is the office staff polite and considerate on the phone and in person? If other parents are in the waiting room, what kind of comments do they make about the doctor? Are they happy with the doctor?

Here are a few other things to consider in meeting your child's special needs:

What are the office hours? Do they meet your schedule needs? If the office is only open a few days a week, then the doctor may not be available when you need him.

Is emergency or after-hours coverage available at all times? You shouldn't be left out in the cold when you need your doctor the most. If the doctor isn't personally available, then who will be covering for her?

Does she have someone who understands children covering her calls? If an internist is covering calls for your doctor, how is that going to help your sick child?

Do nurses or other skilled professionals handle calls after hours? You don't necessarily have to speak to a doctor right away, but you do need to speak to an experienced medical professional who can help guide you to the best next steps. Oftentimes, an experienced nurse can handle almost all the problems that occur after hours. If there is no one who knows children answering calls after hours, then you need to look elsewhere for a doctor to care for your children.

Is there access to specialist care if needed? Not all areas of the country have access to pediatric specialists of various kinds. Hopefully, you'll never need this service, but it's good to know where you can get it if you do.

Here are some other things to ask yourself during the actual interview with a doctor:

- Does the doctor see the parents as partners in the care of their child?
- Does the doctor's personality fit well with your child's?
- Is the doctor a good listener?
- Are you, as a parent, comfortable asking questions to the doctor?
- Is the doctor concerned about preventive care?
- Does the doctor use antibiotics for every cold or respiratory infection or is she more judicious in their use?

Your child's perception of doctors can be shaped for years by his early experiences with the physician you choose. Do your homework. Take the time to research the best doctor for your child.

FINDING A SPECIALIST

Sometimes, despite our best efforts to stay healthy, we get into trouble with a difficult, unusual, or serious medical problem that requires the special training and expertise of a medical specialist. Maybe it's knee replacement surgery, a rare blood disorder, cancer, or heart bypass surgery. Whatever the reason, locating a physician for a specific health need can sometimes be as daunting as the procedures you might face. Where's the best place to start to find a specialist?

The first person to ask when looking for a medical specialist is your primary care doctor. Believe it or not, finding a specialist may be easier than picking your primary care doctor. Why? Because in most cases, you've already got the help of the medical person you trust most . . . your primary care physician.

When you are told that you will need to see a specialist for care, the one question to ask your doctor is, "If you were sick like I am, what doctor would you personally see?" Whoever that person is, get your doctor to get you in to see them for your specialty care—even if it's not in the same town. You need to make it clear that all you want is the best care for your particular medical problem, no matter where it is or what hospital it might be. Here's a good example of what we mean. Your PCP tells you that you have a cancer in your colon and you need surgery. Doctors know that there are fewer complications and better surgical outcomes when colorectal surgeons perform this type of surgery instead of general surgeons. There are many reasons for this, as we'll explain in Chapter 5. They would see the specialist surgeon even if it meant traveling elsewhere for surgery or going to a different hospital.

Next, if there is a particular hospital that you'd like to use, call or get on their Web site and find out what specialists are available in your area of need. Such sites can provide you names of potential candidates. While you have hospital personnel on the phone, ask them about what they've heard about these specialists. What you hear sometimes can be surprising and informative.

Third, go to the American Board of Medical Specialties (ABMS) Web site and look up the doctor's name to make sure he or she is board certified. The site provides information about certification and recertification.

Finally, if you have time, go to interview the specialist much as you would your primary care specialist. Oftentimes, you may not have the luxury of time to conduct interviews because your medical problem requires more immediate action. In these cases, we say trust your doctor. Rarely do you go wrong when you do, especially if she recommends the doctor she would see personally.

Before going to the appointment with the specialist, make sure to gather together all your X rays, blood work, and appropriate medical records and bring them with you. Why? Well, believe it or not, records can get lost when being transferred from one place to another. It's just like when you're drying clothes and two socks go in but mysteriously only one sock comes out when the dryer stops. A doctor's office can be just as mysterious. Records get misplaced on a desk or stuck in a corner. X rays get put in someone else's file. If you take charge and get them yourself, you'll make sure that your specialist has all the information that he or she needs to begin your medical evaluation.

After your consultation with the specialist, ask her to send a note with her findings, diagnosis, and treatment suggestions to your primary care physician. It will provide assurance that your primary physician has all the information he needs to provide the best continuing care for you.

WHAT DOCTORS KNOW ABOUT
Choosing a Doctor and Getting the Best Care . . .
And You Should Too!

---

1. **Don't just ask doctors whom you should go to . . . ask them whom _they_ go to:** Doctors often refer within their own hospitals, networks, or partnerships for business or political reasons. That's good for the hospital or the practice, but not so good for you. There are a lot of group practices with primary care physicians and several specialists who all practice together. What doctors know, and patients don't is that those partnerships are often business- or personal-relationship-based, not

quality-based. What does that mean? It means that they may refer their patients to one another but take their own bodies somewhere else when special care is needed for themselves or their families.

Unless you ask, you'll never know. So next time you ask for a referral and are given one, two, or three names, here's what you need to consider. You might think that the best question to ask would be: "If you were me, which one of these doctors would you go to?" Unfortunately, that is the incorrect question and one that might lead you down a dangerous path.

You are essentially asking the doctor which one of the three referrals he would choose. What would a doctor want to know? "Whom would *you* go to if you had a similar problem?" is the question to ask. And if that doesn't apply for some reason: "Who would you send your mother or father to for care?" No other questions or answers matter as much.

2. **Doctors don't go to doctors that aren't board certified:** There is a joke that every doctor has heard: What do they call the person who graduated last in his class from medical school? *Doctor.* Doctors know that finishing medical school and completing a residency are *not* enough. The best doctors are certified as specialists in their fields. Primary care doctors, like internists or family doctors, should have their board certification just like surgical specialists.

And when you are checking on their board certification, make sure it is one of the twenty-four boards or thirty-six specialties recognized by the American Board of Medical Specialties (ABMS). In some specialties, like plastic surgery, secondary nonaccredited boards have popped up. Don't get these nonaccredited boards confused with real board certification by the ABMS and get a false sense of security. As scary as it might sound, there are doctors practicing who aren't board certified, and in some cases, haven't even finished their residencies. Don't let them practice on you.

The American Board of Medical Specialties (ABMS) publishes

a list of board-certified physicians. The *Official ABMS Directory of Board Certified Medical Specialties* lists doctors names along with their specialty and educational background and is available at most public libraries. You can also go to the ABMS Web site and verify whether or not a physician is board certified at www.abms.org/newsearch.asp. You can also call ABMS at 1-866-ASK-ABMS.

3. **Doctors know that doctors can make mistakes. They speak up and pay attention when they go to the doctor:** Most patients are timid and afraid to ask questions when they go to the doctor. Given how rushed many M.D.s are today, their hurried attitude is almost intended to keep patients quiet and passive.

Many of us get intimidated because of the medical setting. If we were in a restaurant and had been served a bad meal, we'd think nothing of calling the manager over to complain. But in a restaurant, everyone is wearing clothes and standing up. Somehow, when you're lying down wearing a smock that doesn't quite come together in the back and your doctor is standing over you wearing a starched white clinic coat with his name embroidered in blue thread, it isn't an even playing field. In that setting, patients often let doctors treat them like children.

So what do doctors know that you should too? According to a 1999 IOM study, almost 100,000 patients die each year because of errors made by medical personnel. Doctors trust their instincts and you should too. If something doesn't seem or feel right, speak up.

4. **Doctors have other doctors take care of them . . . not their nurse practitioners or their physician's assistants:** Doctors know that going to nurse practitioner school or being trained as a physician's assistant is not the same as going to medical school. Period. In too many health care settings, nurse practitioners and physician's assistants become the in-kind primary care providers—in many instances as a way to keep down staffing costs.

What do doctors know? That practice model is good for the

bottom line of the practice or hospital but not so good for your health and well-being. According to a recent study, women who don't get to consult over the phone with their physician but rather speak to a nurse practitioner are far more likely to be misdiagnosed.

If you call your doctor and ask to speak to him and his nurse calls you instead firmly tell her you want to speak to the doctor. If your doctor does not return your call within twenty-four hours, start looking for a new doctor. That's what your doctor would do.

5. **Doctors know that other doctors are at their best at the start of their day:** Doctors know that as the day wears on, their stress level rises. Unexpected emergencies, procedures taking longer than anticipated—all these surprises make private practice an exercise in "beating the clock" as the day wears on. Doctors know that the more behind they get, the less time they have to answer questions and spend quality time with their patients.

What do doctors know that you should too? Whether scheduling a routine checkup at their primary care physician's office or a major surgery in a hospital, doctors always schedule themselves for the very best care . . . first thing in the morning. This is especially crucial when it comes to surgery. Your surgeon is much more likely to be fresh and rested at the beginning of the day than he is at the end.

Doctors know that hospitals can be a little like airports. Surgeries can get backed up as the day wears on. And doctors know that there is nothing worse than waiting for what seems an eternity for your surgery to begin because your surgeon or the hospital is running behind. Doctors schedule their doctor's visits and surgeries for first thing in the morning . . . and you should too.

6. **Doctors know that getting well and staying healthy is a team effort:** When doctors are in the hands of another colleague, they use a team approach. You'll hear us saying things like, "What are we going to do next?" or "When are we going to get the test results?"

The psychological impact of using *we* and being on the same team as your doctor instead of on the "other side of the treatment table" can make a world of difference in the care you receive. When doctors get care, they put themselves on the team. You should too.

7. **Doctors don't go to doctors who don't explain things well and who get defensive when they are asked questions:** Doctors know that the best doctors are so comfortable with who they are and what they do that they can explain what they do in lay language and with graciousness and charm. When we see a colleague who is belligerent or defensive when we ask questions about care, that is a *huge* red flag that something isn't right. What would a doctor do in the same situation? RUN, RUN, RUN! Take your body somewhere else for your care.

8. **Doctors know that the best doctors don't order a battery of tests until they have taken the time to listen to the patient's concerns and have taken a detailed medical history:** When you watch *ER* or any of the other medical dramas on television, you see residents learning how to take detailed medical histories from their patients before they do anything else for a good reason . . . it works!

    Taking a detailed medical history combined with a comprehensive physical exam is a prerequisite to ordering a battery of tests. Doctors know that some tests are necessary and others aren't. If your doctor starts ordering tests before he has spent time with you, he's not doing a good job and isn't the right person to care for you. (Learn why in Chapter 2.) It could be a sign that he is more concerned about the bottom line of his practice or laboratory income stream than he is about you. Not a good sign and a good reason to find a new doctor.

9. **Doctors know that their doctor has to touch them during a visit:** In many practices, a lot of people—LPNs, RNs, nurse practitioners, physician's assistants, medical assistants—are touching the patients. Unfortunately a lot of doctors are not. Many primary care providers have taken on the role of talk-show host or prescription writer. That just doesn't cut it.

Your doctor has to touch you. Just taking your history and touching your chart with a pen isn't enough. She needs to examine you. She needs to take your temperature, have you say "Aahhh," look down your throat, take a close look and actually touch the area you are worried about. Having a doctor do these simple tasks isn't a luxury, it is the standard of care. Your doctor would expect it, and you should too.

THE BEHIND-THE-SCENES KEY TO GETTING THE BEST CARE IN ANY OFFICE

And now for the bonus round—the insider, insider information about getting the best care that even some doctors tend to miss. The best doctors know that the key to easy, instant access to the best doctors often lies in the hands of the office manager, head nurse, and front office staff.

Many patients think that their HMO or primary care physician is the "gatekeeper" to their health or recovery. Well, this is not even close. Doctors know that the real gatekeepers for the best doctors are their key team members—the office manager and the head nurse. If you make them happy you'll get the very best of everything—the best care, the best appointments, and the best that your doctor has to offer.

Here are our insider tips to being the favorite patient in your doctor's practice:

Come in with a smile (you can be exempt from this in an emergency). Smile and you'll stand out from the crowd immediately.

Learn their names and get to know them. Ask about what they do and are passionate about outside the office.

Bring offerings. It might be something small, like a Starbucks coffee (learn their favorite flavors). A little act of kindness can go a long way.

Say thank you. It's funny, but we probably say thank you more often to the cashier at the grocery store than we do to the people who take care of us and keep us well. Show your thanks in word and deed and your doctor and his team will look forward to your visits and will want to spend more time keeping you healthy and happy. And that might be the most valuable health insurance policy of all!

IS THIS THE RIGHT DOCTOR FOR ME?

When we're interviewing patients for our stories on NBC, we often ask them two questions: "How do you like your doctor?" and "What makes you feel good about your doctor?" After a while, when we looked at the answers, they didn't really surprise us. What they did was provide us with some excellent questions that you might consider asking yourself to evaluate whether or not your doctor is meeting your needs. We believe that many people have a gut feeling about whether or not their physicians are a good fit for them, but haven't formally asked themselves the hard questions. Here are the questions we'd like to see you answer about each of your doctors:

- Does your doctor explain things to you in simple, easy-to-understand terms rather than using medical jargon?

- If she doesn't, can you safely ask her to rephrase the explanation until you can understand it?

- Does your doctor ask you about your concerns or additional question you might have at the end of your appointment?

- Does your doctor make you feel like you are imposing when you ask questions?

- Can you reach your doctor or a nurse when you need advice by phone?

- Does your doctor discuss the side effects of any drug he may prescribe and does he always ask about any other meds or OTC drugs you are taking?

- Does your doctor provide various options for dealing with a medical problem so that you can decide what's best for you?

- When you have problems with an insurance company or managed care organization, will your doctor stand up for you?

- Do you feel comforted after interacting with your doctor?

- If you should be unhappy with your doctor or his staff, do you feel comfortable discussing this with him/her?

Your answers to these questions should help provide some insight into your relationship with your doctor. The doctor-patient relationship should be a partnership. It requires the ability to talk and to listen from both partners. Does your relationship measure up? If not, let your feet do the walking. Get to another doctor who wants to build a relationship, who wants to be a partner in healing with you.

Summary

Finding the right primary care doctor and right specialist is one of the most important things you can do for the overall health of your family. The key is taking this action before an emergency arises and you're forced to deal with a doctor you may or may not like. Interview the doctor you are considering to make sure he's right for you. Good doctors will answer your questions and address your concerns. If you're happy, then your doctor is more likely to be happy as well. The key to the best care is a doctor-patient relationship built on trust.

CHAPTER TWO

THE MEDICAL ENCOUNTER BETWEEN DOCTOR AND PATIENT . . . AND WHAT YOU CAN DO TO HELP

Okay, you've now finished reading Chapter 1, and you've selected a doctor to be your primary care physician or your specialist. That's an important first step, but the actual encounter with the doctor is where the rubber really hits the road. The interaction between doctor and patient is where all the action happens; it's where an actual diagnosis is made and where treatment is rendered. As patients, we are an integral part of what happens in the doctor-patient encounter and we determine in large part the ultimate success of the care we get. We cannot be passive. We must be active participants in our own care. If we're not actively involved in our care, we can easily get the wrong medical care, the wrong diagnosis, and maybe get ourselves killed in the process. The choice is yours.

The encounter between a doctor and a patient can be one of the most rewarding or one of the most frustrating. It helps define the relationship between doctor and patient and sets the tone for all that will happen . . . or will fail to happen. It has to start with making the right diagnosis. If a doctor makes the wrong diagnosis, then he or she will often make the wrong treatment decisions, and we all know what that means—problems for you and for your doctor.

How do you help to shape the medical encounter and make a significant difference in your care? What does a doctor think about as he or she approaches a patient? How does your physician arrive at a diagnosis and how important are you to whatever that final decision is? What questions should you ask *before* going to the doctor's office so that you'll be prepared to get the most out of your visit?

To answer these questions, we'd like to take you behind the scenes and give you an insider's look at how most doctors approach a patient, what the problems are in making a diagnosis, and how you can help in this very difficult process. Hopefully, this chapter will change the way you look at a doctor's visit and help you to understand why each person needs to become a more active participant in the process.

WHAT DOCTORS KNOW ABOUT

Getting the Most Out of the Doctor-Patient Encounter . . . And You Should Too

---

1. The medical encounter requires the active participation of both the doctor and the patient.

2. The best doctors are also great detectives.

3. Taking a history from a patient is the most important part of any medical encounter.

4. Preparing yourself before any visit to a doctor is essential to maximizing the benefits you get from the encounter.

5. You want a doctor who is good at both the art and the science of medicine (we'll clarify exactly what this means later).

6. If you don't trust a doctor, get another. Without trust, there can be no good healing relationship.

THE DOCTOR AS DETECTIVE

Making the correct diagnosis is the most demanding job that a doctor must do. Contrary to what most people would like to believe, medicine is often not black and white, but many shades of gray. Most patients do not present with the classic symptoms of a particular disease. Instead they may have only one or two symptoms of a problem and it is up to the physician to figure out what is going on. It's only when the patient shares all her unique signs and symptoms that a physician can decipher the correct diagnosis from a variety of possibilities.

This is what medicine is all about. The patient must honestly and openly share intimate information with his physician. The physician must listen carefully and apply his or her powers of deduction. It's a two-way street. It takes time and trust, and it takes a doctor with the skills of a detective. He or she must look at the clues and draw certain conclusions based on those clues. Sometimes it's the correct path and sometimes it's not. It takes patience, listening skills, trust by the patient, intuition, and persistence. Making a diagnosis requires sorting through the hundreds of possible things that could be wrong with a person. For many doctors, making the correct diagnosis as quickly as possible with as little inconvenience to the patient is a real point of pride. Getting to the bottom of what is bothering a particular patient is like putting a complicated jigsaw puzzle together. If you're missing a few key pieces, you'll never put the picture together. If the doctor fails to ask a few key questions, or a patient isn't open and honest and doesn't provide the information that's requested, then a piece of the puzzle will be missing, and a diagnosis may be missed, and that could be crucial to one's health.

What doctors attempt to do in any encounter with a patient is to make sure that they don't miss the most serious diseases or diagnosis first. If a patient comes to the doctor complaining of stomach pain that radiates up into the chest at times, the doctor will be most concerned about ruling out heart disease as a possible cause. The doctor knows that these same symptoms could be caused by a problem in a patient's stomach or intestines, but the heart problem is the most serious if missed initially. Doctors will always check for the most serious diseases first and then work backward. This is why you have to have patience with your doctor and allow him or her time to make the correct diagnosis. It may take a few visits and a few tests to do this, but it's all part of being a detective. Different clues take time to check out. After all, it takes Columbo a whole hour to solve a case on TV.

THE IMPORTANCE OF A THOROUGH MEDICAL HISTORY

Studies have shown that doctors can make a diagnosis 70 to 80 percent of the time simply by taking a good history from the patient. The key to good patient care is asking the right questions, listening carefully to what is said both verbally and nonverbally, and then, and only then, examining the patient.

When learning how to take care of people, medical students learn what is called a "review of systems"—an in-depth, detailed review of all body systems using many, many questions. Not only should this include a review of the body from head to toe but also a family history, social history, personal habits like smoking and alcohol use, sexual history, occupational history, past medical history, and a medication history. The purpose behind all these questions is to help define a patient's potential medical problems in the hope of refining what laboratory and other tests are needed to come to a diagnosis.

Sure, it's easy to bombard someone with a wide variety of tests, but that doesn't provide an accurate picture of their health—the health of a person's integrated mind, body, and spirit. This can only be obtained after a doctor takes the time to sit down and carefully take a medical history. A good history is almost like having someone tell their doctor the story of their life. Your doctor will not take a complete history on every visit, but if your primary care doctor never asks for all your health information, find someone else. Specialists don't necessarily need all this information, but they too should take a history, with a particular focus on their specialty area.

The problem that many doctors face—and the one that patients complain about the most—is the lack of time available for each patient. Managed care organizations push physicians to be more productive in their quest for profits, so there isn't as much time allowed for encounters with patients. So what suffers? History taking suffers, which means the ability to make the correct diagnosis is hurt as well. And of course it also means that every one of us who is a patient suffers. What can you do to help? You can prepare yourself prior to your visit so that you get the most out of your encounter with your doctor in whatever time you have.

The key to helping your doctor make the right diagnosis is providing the best answers to your doctor's questions. Here's how you can help:

Ten Tips to Help Your Doctor Make the Correct Diagnosis

1. **Think about your problem prior to seeing your doctor and write down all the pertinent facts so you don't forget the most important things.** It's hard to believe, but when patients come in to see us, they are often confused about their problem or act unsure of the

Kevin's Comments

During my years in the emergency room, there was nothing more frustrating than to see a patient with a rambling story and a variety of complaints. My biggest problem was trying to figure out why they really came to the ER. I always believed that for most people to come to the ER to be seen, something had changed or was bothering them enough to make a difference in their life. My job was to figure out what that was. I always wished that these patients had thought out what their real goal was for that ER visit. It would have made them a lot happier, and saved me a lot of time, tests, and heartburn.

signs and symptoms they have. It's easy to become confused if you are seeing a doctor who appears rushed, who is peppering you with questions, and who is out the door before you can clear your head. Write your concerns down before you come in for your visit. We've all had the experience of being halfway home and suddenly remembering an important question you wanted to ask your doctor. Then, the only way to get it answered is to start playing phone tag with the office. Remember, write down your concerns. It's the only way you won't forget what's most important to you.

2. **Decide what the key issues are that you want addressed and prioritize them.** If you had one main issue that you wanted addressed, what would it be? We've seen patients with multiple, vague complaints that are all over the map. You can't possibly address them all in a single visit, especially if you're scheduled for a ten-minute office visit. If you have multiple problems, then consider scheduling more time with your doctor. Prioritize your concerns and get the most important ones addressed at the beginning of the visit. If all your concerns aren't addressed, make another appointment to see your physician soon.

3. **Think about your symptoms—when did they begin, how long do they last, and what makes them better or worse.** These are the questions that a good doctor will be asking and focusing on when he speaks with you. Think about them ahead of time so that you can provide the best possible answers. "What makes your problem better or worse?" is one of the most important questions and will help focus the doctor in terms of potential testing. If, for instance, your headache is relieved by an OTC medicine and seems to occur when you are under stress, that helps the doctor to know that it's not likely a brain tumor, so an MRI test is not indicated on that first visit.

4. **Tell your story succinctly and let your doctor ask questions to clarify your concerns.** Keep it short and sweet. This is a good rule of thumb for us all when giving our history. If you ramble without being

focused, it's difficult for the doctor to concentrate on your most important problem. Trust us, doctors will ask you questions to get the kind of information that they need. Highlight the most important facts, and then let the doctor ask you about the details he or she needs.

5. **Don't be afraid to tell your doctor about the signs and symptoms that are bothering you, even if he doesn't specifically ask about them.** If you are interrupted in recounting your story, as physicians are prone to do, or you suddenly remember some important problem you forgot to mention, make sure to tell your doctor, as it can be extremely important. It just might be that last piece of the jigsaw puzzle that they need to complete the picture of your specific medical illness. If it's important to you, then it should be important to them.

6. **Do mention anything that is different about you since your last visit, as the change could be related to your medical problem or to a medicine you are taking.** If something changes in your condition or how you feel since your last visit or since you began taking a new medicine, tell your doctor. Clare was a friend of Kevin's who began taking a medicine for hypertension and shortly afterward developed a cough. She mentioned it to him one day and he told her that this particular medicine had a very common side effect of causing a cough. She had just seen her doctor, but she had failed to mention the problem. She called the doctor the next day. He switched her blood pressure medicine and the cough immediately disappeared. Tell your doctor about any changes in your health since your last visit. He isn't a mind reader and may fail to ask you specifically about particular health symptoms that may have changed since you began a specific medicine or treatment. Also, since many of us see more than one doctor, your doctor won't be able to remember or refer to something he doesn't even know about. All of your doctors need to know about all of the medicine you are taking and the treatments that you are undergoing.

7. **List all the medications and supplements you are taking.** Write them down on a piece of paper—names and dosages—and bring it with you to your doctor visit. We suggest keeping a copy in your wallet as well, just in case of an emergency. Too many patients do not know the names of the medication they take . . . they can't even describe the color or shape of the pills, or what they are taking the medication for. It's vital that you have a list of all the medicine you are taking. We can't emphasize this point enough.

   We've seen and heard about too many situations in which the patient doesn't tell the doctor about everything else they're taking. Your doctor may order tests to pursue a problem that's caused by some herbal supplement or some OTC medicine that you're taking. Here's a good example: One of our friends was taking ephedra, an herbal supplement that supposedly provides more energy. She went to the doctor for help sleeping. So the doctor gave her some sleeping pills that produced some very bad side effects. She decided on her own to stop all her medicines and supplements. Sure enough, all her problems resolved. If her doctor had known that she was taking ephedra, he would likely have told her first to stop taking that before trying any sleep medications. In this case, it might have avoided some serious unwanted side effects.

8. **Be honest about the level of pain that occurs during the physical examination. Downplaying this may cause the doctor to underestimate your problem.** Pain is an important symptom for a doctor. It tells us that something is wrong and we'd better look more closely at what's going on. It helps to guide our examination, diagnosis, and treatment. If you went to the ER with a complaint of abdominal pain and then downplayed your symptoms, it might mislead the doctor into thinking that you had a simple case of gastritis when in fact you had appendicitis, a condition requiring surgery before the appendix bursts. Don't be a hero. If it hurts, let your doctor know it.

9. **Don't wait until the doctor is leaving the room before mentioning a particular concern you have, or the problem might not get the attention it deserves.** This is something that really frustrates doctors. Several times a day, our patients because of embarrassment or hesitation don't tell us the thing they are most concerned about until we are saying goodbye and are about to walk them out of the treatment room.

   Here's how it goes: The doctor goes into a room to examine a patient. He makes his diagnosis and write a prescription. He's heading out the door when the patient mentions something that completely alters the way he's thought about the problem or leads him to an even more important problem. Thank goodness that something has been said, but the patient shouldn't wait until the end of the visit to mention a problem.

10. **Be sure to tell your doctor if you'd had something like this previously or what you think your problem may be. Patients are often right.** Good doctors like to hear what you think your problem might be. It helps them in their thinking and will help them to address your specific concerns. If your doctor is unwilling to listen to you, find another doctor.

   Patients are often correct in guessing what they may have, and it just may be something that your doctor hasn't thought about. Oftentimes, if you've had something like this previously, you'll know what's wrong or what's been successful or unsuccessful in treating this in the past.

Taking the time to think about your visit before you go to the doctor can pay huge dividends. Why not? After all, it's your health that's on the line.

THE ART OF MEDICINE

To be a really good doctor, a physician must master two very different disciplines—one is the science of medicine and the other is the art of medicine. The science of medicine involves all the scientific or technical information that is needed to practice medicine. It involves a tremendous amount of highly detailed scientific knowledge encompassing a wide variety of medical disciplines.

The art of medicine concerns the interaction between doctor and patient and requires the ability to speak to patients in a style that maximizes communication. Ideal communication requires a dialogue or exchange of information between two people. The best physicians, those skilled in the art of medicine, understand that they must listen to the story that people want and

Kevin's Comments

Phil was a patient whom I saw one night in the ER. He was a smoker with a one-week history of a cough. Because he had a fever and some crackles in his chest when I examined him, I ordered a chest X ray. It was normal and showed no pneumonia or other abnormalities. I told Phil that he had a simple case of bronchitis and I prescribed some medicines for him. I didn't know it, but Phil was really concerned that he might have lung cancer. He didn't say anything to me about his concern and I certainly did not specifically say anything about not seeing cancer on his X ray before I left him. Fortunately, he mentioned his concern to my nurse and so I was able to go back in and calm his fears.

If you have a specific medical problem that you're worried about, please let your doctor know so that he or she can address it directly. Doctors aren't mind readers, and almost any doctor I've ever known wants to do a good job and have their patients leave happy and satisfied.

need to tell, if the patient is to be served at the highest possible level. It requires a doctor who is kind, sensitive, caring, seems to have time for patients, and listens to what they are trying to say. We believe that these attributes are what distinguish the excellent physicians from the average ones.

Being a master of the art of medicine also requires an understanding of the cultural diversity of the people the physician serves. It also demands the ability to listen to what the patient is saying both formally and informally. Unfortunately, despite the obvious importance of these skills, medical schools give little time or attention to helping medical students master them. As a result, we may have to help continue the education of our doctors as we go to them for care.

Physicians must, in a fifteen-minute visit, determine symptoms, make diagnoses, get to know the patient's psychosocial situation, develop a therapeutic relationship, and counsel the patient about behaviors and therapies. Could anyone possibly meet these kinds of demands? Yet this is what we ask of physicians all the time. Doctors definitely can use our help because we don't know one yet who can meet our expectations without our help, but it takes a great deal of trust on our part.

DO YOU TRUST YOUR DOCTOR?

Taking a few minutes after you visit your doctor's office to answer some simple questions will provide invaluable insight into the level of trust and confidence that you have in her. If the majority of the answers to the questions are negative, are you willing to "keep on getting what you're getting" or are you ready to be proactive and take charge so that you, and your family, get the health care you want and deserve?

Here are some questions we think you need to answer after every doctor visit:

- Do you think your doctor will do whatever it takes to get you all the care you need?

■ Do you believe your doctor only thinks about what is best for you?

■ Are his or her medical skills current and what you expect?

■ Is your doctor both thorough and careful?

■ Does your doctor pay full attention to you when you are telling your story?

■ Does your doctor provide you with all your treatment options for your particular medical problem?

■ Do you trust your doctor's medical staff to tell you the truth and to look after your best interests?

■ Are you willing to put your life in your doctor's hands? (Because this what you are doing.)

When you walk away from each medical encounter, you'd better think about these questions because if you don't trust your doctor, you're in trouble and you need to find another one. Trust is at the cornerstone of the doctor-patient relationship.

BEGIN WITH THE END IN MIND

Stephen Covey, in his bestselling book, *The Seven Habits of Highly Effective People*, urges people to "Begin with the end in mind." This is great advice. So, what kind of relationship do you want with your doctor or health care professional? You have to know what you want before you can get it. You have to have a goal in mind. You have to know how you want to feel, and be prepared to act if you don't get what you need. As in any other relationship, changing the doctor-patient relationship takes time and energy. You have to be honest and open in what your needs are and then work to communicate these needs to your doctor . . . one visit at a time. If you don't say anything, then your doctor will assume everything's all right.

Here's a great story to illustrate our point. One of our friends in Texas took his elderly father to see an orthopedist in a nearby larger city because his dad had knee pain and it seemed to be worsening. They had an appointment at 10 A.M. in the morning but weren't brought back to the doctor's exam room until after eleven. About fifteen minutes later, a nurse came in and asked the reason for the visit and several more questions. Finally, about a half hour later, the same nurse and the doctor came back in. The doctor listened to the nurse for a couple of minutes, asked one question of our friend's dad, and then told him that he'd give him an injection in his knee to make him feel better. He then told the nurse to get things ready and he'd be back in a couple of minutes. The doctor returned about ten minutes later (about two and a half hours after the scheduled appointment), injected the knee, and then told the elderly man that he'd like to see him in about six weeks. He then turned to leave.

Now this is where the story begins to be fun. The son, a very mild-mannered man, stopped the doctor at the door and told him that he'd like to ask him a couple of questions. The doctor agreed. The son pointed at all the degrees and certificates hanging on the wall in the room and then asked the doctor if his time was very important to him. The doctor, of course, said that it was. The dialogue then went something like this:

Son: *I bet you enjoy going out to dinner sometimes don't you, Doctor?*
Doctor: *Yes, I go with my family sometimes and other times just with my wife.*
Son: *Do you make reservations sometimes because you don't want to have to wait too long at a restaurant?*
Doctor: *Sure I do, my time is pretty important to me, and I don't like having to wait for no good reason.*
Son: *I don't blame you. What happens when you get to that restaurant where you have a reservation and they don't sit you down for an hour or so after your reservation? Are you upset, angry, and seriously consider whether or not you'll ever go back there again?*
Doctor: *Of course I am. But what's the point of all these questions? I'm really busy today.*

Son: The point is that my father and I had an appointment and still waited for two and a half hours before seeing you, and then only briefly, with almost no explanation on your part. I don't think this is the way you'd like to be treated.

According to our friend, the doctor immediately got that lightbulb-going-off look on his face and then smiled. He quickly apologized for how the son and his father were treated and told them that it was a good lesson for him. He then sat down and asked if either of them had any more questions. When all the questions were answered, the doctor wrote down his nurse's phone number and told them to make sure to call her before the next appointment so that he could make sure he did better about getting them seen at the appointed time.

Our point to each of you: You have to ask for the kind of service or care that you want. Sometimes people continue to act in a certain way because they think they are doing a good job. Why should they change what they're doing or how they're acting if no one has complained? What should be your responsibility as a good patient in all this?

You must learn to speak up if you aren't treated properly, if you aren't listened to, if you are treated rudely by the physician or his/her staff, if you aren't treated with respect, or if you don't understand what is being said to you. It's only when we confront a situation that there is any chance for change to occur. If we keep our feelings, thoughts, and emotions inside, we are to blame if nothing changes. No one can read our minds, least of all a busy, time-driven doctor with many patients to see. We must take responsibility for ourselves and take constructive action to get what we want.

CONSTRUCTIVE STEPS FOR GETTING WHAT YOU NEED

So, how do we confront a health care professional (or for that matter, anyone else) about their unacceptable behavior? Clearly, we don't do it by yelling angrily, becoming hostile, speaking nastily, or treating the person with disrespect. If we do, it's the surest way to put someone immediately on the defensive, not get heard, and last but not least, not get what we want. Therefore, we must confront calmly and in a manner that will get people's attention. Here are some steps that will get you what you want and need, and let the other person feel good at the same time:

Talk about your feelings: Tune in to what's going on inside yourself emotionally and state what you are feeling. "I feel (*state how you feel*)." "I feel angry inside because (*state the reason*)." "I feel very dissatisfied because the doctor didn't answer my questions and I've been waiting for two hours (*or whatever the reason is*)."

State the reason behind your feeling: "I feel angry because your receptionist was extremely rude when I asked her why I had not been seen when my appointment was over an hour ago. I feel very dissatisfied with this visit because you never once looked at me and you never listened to me for more than a few seconds before interrupting."

Explain what you would like to see happen or change: I would like to speak to your receptionist with you present and then receive an apology if appropriate after I hear her story. I would like for you to spend more time with me so that you can listen to my primary complaint more fully.

Listen to the other side of the story and be willing to negotiate: There are always two sides to a story. Listen to the other person's story and then negotiate based on what you heard. In our examples, the receptionist may say that she had just gotten word that her mother was very ill or that she had just been treated badly by someone on the phone. She admitted that she was short-tempered and it was her fault. Enough said. The doctor may say that he really is listening but that he's afraid that looking directly at people makes them uncomfortable. You definitely can negotiate this one.

Define the consequences if things don't change to your liking: "If we can't negotiate a settlement that is satisfactory to me, then I will take my business elsewhere, state my dissatisfaction to my friends, and write the managed care plan to which I belong of my unhappiness and the reason why."

The biggest weapon that we possess as patients is our ability to walk and talk with our pocketbooks. If doctors don't have patients, then they don't make money, don't get to operate, don't get to enjoy the euphoria of making an astute diagnosis or maybe even saving a life, and don't get the "emotional income" they need from you the patient. If your doctor can't or is unwilling to meet a reasonable demand, then consider going elsewhere for your care.

It's a commonly accepted fact that a dissatisfied customer will tell ten other people about his or her bad experience, while satisfied customers may tell one other person. If enough patients speak up verbally and/or with their purse strings, a poor physician will ultimately feel the impact and maybe, just maybe, change his or her behavior, but only if he or she is told about the problem.

Finally, certain doctors may not be for you . . . or for anyone else. Here are a few warning signs that should tell you that it's time to look for another doctor.

- Evades questions

- Doesn't explain your diagnosis or treatment

- Never apologizes for being late

- Is rude

- Is hours late for appointment time—constantly

- Never lays hands on you during an exam

- Makes sexual advances

- Acts unethically

- Is reluctant to change a treatment plan even when faced with other evidence

If you have any of these problems or issues with your doctor, run—don't walk—out of the door. If you have sexual issues or ethical concerns about a doctor, we strongly suggest reporting him or her to your state board of medical examiners and let them investigate your concerns. A conspiracy of silence doesn't help anyone. We need to trust our doctors before we can share the most intimate aspects of our lives and, literally, place our lives in their hands.

IMPROVING THE QUALITY OF MEDICAL CARE

There is no doubt that the American health care system is among the best in the world. One need only visit the best hospitals in America on any given day and you will find both doctors and patients from all over the world giving or receiving care. Why? The U.S. system of health care is the most technically advanced in the world and we have the equipment to make the best diagnoses and provide the highest quality of treatment. We also spend more money on health care than any other country in the world. But the U.S. system is not without problems. One example: Despite all we spend on health care, our infant mortality rate (death rate of our youngest children) is not even among the five lowest in the world. Despite all the money thrown at it, our present system of health care often does not deliver on the care that it promises or knows to be good.

In late 1999, the Institute of Medicine (IOM) issued an in-depth report entitled *To Err is Human* that defines the critical defects in the United States system of health care. The report states that ninety thousand lives could be saved annually if deficiencies in patient safety were corrected. In March 2001, the IOM published *Crossing the Quality Chasm* which cited an urgent need to improve patient safety as well as addressing concerns related to the timely delivery of care, the efficiency of care, and equity in care. The 2001 IOM report noted that poor-quality health care was not confined to any one group but was pervasive throughout the system, found at all levels of care—acute, chronic, and preventive—and affected even those with access to the best doctors and hospitals.

Quality problems in health care are not new. In the 1970s, researchers noted unexplained differences in the areas of surgical procedures and hospital admissions from one geographic area to the next. Since then, variations in clinical practice patterns have been widely documented. Even though medicine is a science and you would think that science is fairly exact, medical care can vary widely from doctor to doctor and from place to place. Contrary to what we may want to believe, the quality of medical care is anything but uniform and patients do not always get the most appropriate medical treatment. The obvious question is: "If something is good for a certain group of patients, then why don't all doctors follow that practice?" The only answer to this is: "There is no good reason." This is why many physicians and medical organizations are urging the adoption and use of what's know in medicine as evidence-based guidelines for the best practice of medicine.

EVIDENCE-BASED MEDICINE

In 1989, a new federal agency, the Agency for Health Care Policy and Research, was created, and one of the tasks that it was given was the creation and promotion of medical practice guidelines. The hope by the legislature was that explicit guidelines would be a mechanism for promoting a specific standard of care.

The idea was to take what had been learned in clinical trials and research and translate that information into recommendations for the treatment of all other patients with a similar condition—to take a treatment that has been proven to be effective, beneficial, and safe and then provide that information to physicians so that they can use it for the benefit of their patients when appropriate.

In evidence-based medicine (EBM), guidelines are set up to help limit inappropriate care, decrease the magnitude of geographic variations in the way doctors practice, and ensure that health care resources are used for the maximum benefit of patients. Practice guidelines are a way of ensuring a certain level of quality in medicine as well as helping to reduce the risk of malpractice. This, in a nutshell, is evidence-based medicine. Sounds great, doesn't it? How can anyone complain about having something like this in his or her clinical arsenal?

There are concerns raised by a number of doctors that EBM is a ploy by insurers or managed care organizations to deny payment for treatments unless it has been proven beyond doubt that it works. (Trust us, nothing in medicine works all the time in every patient). However, EBM advocates prefer that providers *not* provide treatments to patients that have been shown to be ineffective, harmful, or to have poor value.

There's an old axiom: "Raise the water level so all ships rise." That perhaps is what EBM is meant to do. If you raise the levels of care by providing standards of best care for the medical community, then all patients will ultimately benefit.

Here are a few examples of evidence-based medical care that all patients should receive and why:

Beta-blocking drugs after heart attacks: Beta blockers are heart drugs that should be administered to patients shortly after a heart attack. If patients get these cardiac drugs, their chances of dying and of having a second heart attack are greatly reduced. (Only about one-third of patients now get this after heart attacks despite its proven benefit.)

Aspirin in a heart attack: Aspirin helps reduce the chances of blood clotting. Research has shown that giving the equivalent of a baby aspirin on the first day of a heart attack and continuing this for a month can reduce the chances of dying by almost 25 percent. The latest research indicates that taking "super" aspirin for a year will reduce the risk of death by almost 40 percent, yet many patients are not told of aspirin's benefit after a heart attack.

ACE inhibitors in heart failure: Drugs known as angiotensin-converting enzymes (ACE inhibitors) should be used in patients with heart failure because they reduce the risk of dying by one-quarter. These drugs also lessen the chances of the heart failure worsening. Again, many patients are not put on these medications, as they should be in the case of heart failure.

Want another example of evidence-based guidelines for best practice? If you have high blood pressure, a wide variety of medicines can be used to bring it back to a normal range. Certain well-respected government agencies have issued clear-cut guidelines on how to treat blood pressure using a very specific step-by-step approach. If you are mildly hypertensive (elevated blood pressure) and you are a white female with no other diseases, then you should begin with a certain type of medicine. If you are a black male, then you should likely begin with another type of medicine. It's a straightforward and easy-to-follow guideline for all doctors. So if this is the case, then why do researchers find that only 23 percent of all patients with high blood pressure have their blood pressure under control? Part of the reason is that doctors aren't following the clearly defined guidelines. (Another factor is that patients aren't complying with the care their doctor has prescribed, something we'll discuss later.)

So what's the problem? Why don't doctors take advantage of these guidelines and provide medicines that can help save patients lives, especially when they've been proven effective? Many factors prevent these evidence-based guidelines from being incorporated into clinical practice in the real world. First, managed care and the requirements of a busy practice limit the time that doctors have with each patient. Second, keeping up with the latest research and best clinical treatments requires extensive time and effort because there is so much research published. Third, nobody likes to change their old way of doing things even if medical practice has changed.

We can't stress this last point enough. There are numerous well-documented instances in clinical practice (and many examples that we've seen for ourselves) in which the practice of medicine has passed physicians by or new physicians have not been taught to practice medicine that is supported by the clinical data like that utilized in evidence-based medicine. Despite guidelines issued by national organizations, compliance with EBM is distressingly low.

As consumers of medical care, we should expect that our physicians would participate in the practice of EBM. Why? Simply put, medicine is just too complicated for the unassisted human mind. Just because a physician believes something to be true about medical care doesn't make it so. Medicine needs to be based on empirical data. There is so much new information and research published every year that physicians cannot possibly keep up. For instance, what doctor can possibly know seventeen thousand medicines, their side effects, and their interactions with other prescription drugs, much less OTC meds or herbal supplements. It's not a failing on their part. It's reality. No one can do it. So what's should each of us be doing?

We cannot assume that our individual physician has done the right thing. Medicine is just too complex. Doctors need help. You can ask your doctor if she uses evidence-based medicine when appropriate. If she answers yes, then great. But if not, you should ask, "why not?" We then urge you to look up information about EBM at www.guidelines.gov. There are currently more than nine hundred medical practice guidelines, and this site provides information on all of them. Be aware of your condition and make sure that the best evidence doesn't conflict with your doctor's treatment plan for you. If it does, ask your doctor about the difference and ask him or her to explain the reasons for their different approach. If you are not satisfied with the answer, seek a second opinion.

Summary

To gain the most from the doctor-patient relationship, it takes the active participation of both doctors and patients. Think about what you want from the relationship and work toward the end you have in mind. Finally, do your medical research, as there is just too much at stake. Doctors know that they don't know it all . . . and you should too.

CHAPTER THREE

MEDICAL TESTING AND SCREENING: WHAT KIND OF TESTS TO GET AND WHEN

Do you ever wonder why doctors run the kinds of tests they do? Is there some pattern or reason why people get some tests and not others? Do you ever wonder what tests doctors want done on themselves when they go for their medical exam?

Medical testing is a relatively new phenomenon that came into being in the twentieth century. Prior to this time, doctors had only one or two medical tests that they could offer to their patients. It was extremely frustrating. Even if testing had been available, there was little treatment that doctors could offer in the way of actual medications until around the time of World War II when huge advances in pharmaceuticals began to occur.

Now, thanks to advances in technology, there is almost no part of the human body that can't be tested. But just because we can test, should we test? Is the cost of performing certain tests justified? Should testing for women be different than it is for men? We'll explore these questions and many more in this chapter. The answers may surprise you, and hopefully will change the kind of tests you ask your doctor to perform in order to keep you healthy.

MEDICAL SCREENING

Bear with us for a minute. We're going to give you a little medical history lesson because it's important for your understanding of how we got to where we are today in the medical testing and medical screening of most people.

Back in the 1950s, the medical community embraced the concept of multiphasic health screening—i.e., doctors performed a variety of medical tests on everyone no matter what the status of their health. It was the era of "executive" or annual physicals in which healthy-appearing persons received electrocardiograms, chest X rays, blood tests of every kind, and urine testing. Little or nothing was ever found, but it seemed like a good idea. How could anyone possibly find fault with doing more tests? After all, the more diagnostic tests one administers, the healthier we will be and the longer we will live. (This is not true, but it was the belief at the time.)

This trend continued into the seventies when scientists began to question the wisdom of all this testing on people. Was all this testing really improving people's health and enabling them to live longer and better lives? Did it generate false positives that needed to be explored and then create more problems for the patient when further tests were done? Had our ability to test outpaced our ability as doctors to understand what the data really meant?

It took a number of epidemiology studies in the late seventies to debunk the assumptions behind this large-scale multiphasic health testing. Epidemi what? Let us explain. Epidemiology is the field of medical science that studies the causes and determinants of disease in large populations of people. Epidemiology is an extremely important tool in our understanding of how various lifestyles, jobs, or exposures impact our health. It was epidemiologists who discovered the link between asbestos exposure and lung cancer as well as the link between smoking and lung cancer.

In the studies involving medical testing, scientists compared the disease rate (morbidity) and the death rate (mortality) in those undergoing screening compared to groups of people who didn't have the "advantage" of screening. They even did this in people who had disease versus those who didn't. What they found was that **screening had little, if any, impact on the overall health of those going through this expensive multiphasic health testing.** One of the more famous studies done in the 1970s was known as the South-East London Screening Study. In it, the authors concluded the following: "Since these controlled trial results have failed to demonstrate any beneficial effect on either mortality or morbidity, we believe that the use of general practice based multiphasic screening in the middle aged can no longer be advocated on scientific, ethical, or economic grounds as a desirable public health measure."

This was an extremely powerful statement and rocked conventional thinking. It took a few more years of study, but finally, in 1985, the AMA stated in the *Journal of the American Medical Association* that, "Unfortunately, the early enthusiasm was clearly overstated. Multiphasic screening turned out to be a mixed blessing."

Big deal. So the medical community tried all this testing and found it to be unnecessary for the general healthy population. Surely, then, these screening programs would provide better value if used for specific high-risk populations like smokers or those with liver disease. The National Cancer Institute (NCI) thought the same thing and decided to conduct a few studies to test this hypothesis.

The NCI knew that smokers were more at risk for cancer than the general population. Theoretically, if you could detect cancer, you might help people get treatment sooner and, as a result, live longer. In the 1980s, a number of health studies were done to see if cigarette smokers who had regular chest X rays or sputum cytologies (examination of lung cells found in the mucus that people coughed up) lived longer than those who were not tested regularly. Believe it or not, to the surprise of almost all the experts, those who received frequent screenings and frequent chest X rays lived no longer and did no better than those who weren't screened. Physicians were shocked at these findings and often found it difficult to explain to patients why they stopped doing certain kinds of tests. These studies were the precise reason why doctors stopped doing annual chest X rays. Patients would often say, "Why aren't you giving me a chest X ray? I've gotten one for years." It's very difficult for a doctor to say, "I'm not doing a chest X ray on you because the data shows that it's often too late to do anything by the time a tumor shows up on the X ray." Not very reassuring, is it?

Similarly, a group of patients with hepatitis were regularly screened for liver cancer because they had a 150 percent increased risk of contracting cancer compared to persons without any liver problems. Surprisingly, those screened received no real benefit over those not screened. These two examples well illustrate the point that not all testing is worthwhile. The lesson to all of us: The testing we do today may change with time as we conduct more studies. We may add some tests based on new data and we may delete others. Change is inevitable, so we shouldn't be surprised.

SCREENING TESTS: WHAT DO DOCTOR'S RECOMMEND FOR MEN AND WOMEN?

Mrs. Mealia is a forty-two-year-old woman who comes to her doctor's office asking for a complete physical examination. She has no particular health concerns but has read lately that everyone should have a complete physical annually. She works for a company where the top managers get physicals every year. Her doctor tells her that she only needs a few simple tests and not to waste her money getting a complete battery of tests. He explains that taking a shotgun approach is just not good medicine anymore and that it increases costs without real benefit. Mrs. Mealia feels like her doctor doesn't care and, because she's in an HMO, wonders if cost concerns are the entire reason behind why her doctor doesn't recommend more testing. She's now trying to decide whether or not to switch to another physician.

Now we're getting to the heart of the matter for most people. Because annual visits to the doctor were pushed so aggressively in the past, there is now a great deal of confusion about how often a person should be tested and what tests are needed. One of the questions that we hear over and over again from friends and patients is, **"With all the possible medical tests out there, and some of them pretty darn expensive, how do I know which ones are best for me?"** This is the bottom line: What tests are useful? Which ones are a waste of time or provide very little cost benefit for most people?

It would be great if we had all the money in the world to spend on testing, but we, as a country, and most of us individually, don't have that luxury. So how can we maximize the benefit of the tests that we do get? It's really very simple, and the best medical minds in the country look at this question on a regular basis as part of the United States Preventive Services Task Force. The USPSTF looks at all the possible tests and recommends which tests are best for most people, considering cost, ability to diagnose, and the ability to detect before a disease causes severe damage to a person's health. (You can look at their recommendations at www.ahcpr.gov/clinic/prevenix.)

Based on the USPSTF recommendations, doctors suggest certain medical tests because they will reveal where most people will have problems, and

Major Causes of Death in the United States

Men's Health Risks	Women's Health Risks
1. Heart disease	1. Heart disease
2. Cancer	2. Cancer
3. Accidents and adverse effects	3. Stroke
4. Stroke	4. Chronic obstructive pulmonary disease
5. Chronic obstructive pulmonary disease	5. Pneumonia and influenza
6. Pneumonia and influenza	6. Diabetes
7. Diabetes	7. Accidents and adverse effects

if they pick up these problems early enough, they can make a clear difference in the people's lives and their state of health.

If you look at the table of the major reasons why men and women die, you will see that they are very similar. What's different is the order of each. So why wouldn't we focus our screening efforts on those diseases that cause men and women the most problems? In fact, we do. Here are the screening tests we consider the most important. (We didn't arrive at this solely by ourselves but consulted some of the top medical organizations and groups in the country to arrive at our list.)

Essential Medical Tests for Males

1. Blood Pressure Test

High blood pressure (or hypertension) is known as the "silent killer." Most of us have no symptoms when our blood pressure is high. The longer high blood pressure goes undetected and untreated, the greater the risk of heart attack, stroke, heart failure, and kidney damage for both men and women. A blood pressure test should be done at least every two years when you're younger but annually over the age of forty. We're more conservative than many others when it comes to checking your pressure.

People with diabetes, who are overweight, or who have a family history of diabetes are at greatest risk for blood pressure problems and should be checked more frequently. African-Americans are more at risk for hypertension at earlier ages than whites, so they should be checked annually at a younger age.

Ideally, according to the latest guidelines, we should keep our systolic (top number) below 120 and our diastolic (lower number) below 80 (see the classifications and guidelines in Chapter 8). Hypertension begins at 140 systolic and 90 diastolic and should be treated, especially if a person is diabetic or has kidney disease.

2. Colon Examination *(see the chapter on cancer for more details)*

Colorectal cancer is a cancer that is largely preventable with frequent exams. A fecal occult blood test is often used as a screening test, but by age fifty, a colonoscopy should be done. If your test is normal, you don't have to have another one for three to five years. If you're at higher risk for colon cancer because of family history, the test should be done at an earlier age and more frequently.

3. **Prostate Screening Exam** *(see the chapter on cancer for more details)*

The prostate gland enlarges as we age, and by fifty, about half of men have a noncancerous condition called benign prostatic hypertrophy (BPH). A digital rectal exam will find this condition or men will notice that their plumbing doesn't work as well. We recommend annual PSA blood tests beginning at age fifty unless a man is at high risk for prostate cancer.

4. **Skin Examination**

Skin cancer is the most common cancer in the United States, and those at greatest risk are those who have had the most sun exposure over the years. Most skin cancers can be removed before they cause further health problems. You should expect a complete skin examination at the time of your regular full physical examination. This is especially important for people over age forty because skin damage begins to show up in later years.

5. **Cholesterol Tests** *(see the chapter on cardiovascular disease for more details)*

You notice that we said tests and not a single test. Total cholesterol is an inadequate assessment of the impact of cholesterol on your arteries. Your doctor needs to measure HDL, LDL, and triglycerides as well. Only then can you know the risk you may have from cholesterol. Examinations should begin in your twenties and then take place every three to five years unless you have elevated levels of cholesterol.

6. **C-Reactive Protein Test** *(see the chapter on cardiovascular disease for more details)*

This is one of the newest tests that doctors are ordering and is a measure of inflammation in the body. Those with elevated levels of CRP are at increased risk for heart attacks and stroke. There are many different conditions that can elevate CRP and most are correctable. Tests should begin at age thirty and be repeated at the same time interval as cholesterol level testing.

7. Dental Examination

Although there are no firm guidelines from the CDC (Centers for Disease Control) on how often adults should get dental exams, for maximum oral health, you should see your dentist at least once a year for a comprehensive dental examination and at least twice a year for a cleaning of your teeth and gums. Many adults need to have periodontal (gum) cleanings more often than every six months—for many, once every three to four months is what is needed in order to keep your teeth and gums healthy and free of infection and disease.

Regular visits to the dentist can help:

- Prevent tooth decay.

- Prevent or treat gum disease (also known as periodontal disease).

- Prevent periodontal disease, which has been associated with increased risk of coronary artery disease and peripheral vascular disease, placing people at risk for heart attack or stroke.

- Prevent bacterial infections of the gums.

At least, twice-yearly dental visits are especially important if you:

- Have diabetes, since poor control of insulin levels can result in gum disease.

- Smoke, since tobacco makes gum disease worse.

- Are pregnant, since hormonal changes are associated with gingivitis, a condition in which the gums become red and swollen.

■ Take prescription or over-the-counter medications that reduce saliva (and make your mouth feel dry), placing individuals at risk for cavities and gum disease.

8. Urinalysis

Urine tests can detect the presence of infection. Red blood cells in the urine can signify a tumor or problems with your kidneys or bladder. Tests should take place during every routine complete examination or if symptoms suggest problems.

9. Complete Blood Count (CBC)

The CBC measures how well your bone marrow and immune system is working. It measures white blood cells (indicative of infection), hemoglobin and hematocrit (indicative of the ability of the blood to carry oxygen and the presence of anemia), and platelets (indicative of the clotting ability of the blood). It can help detect disorders of the blood. It is not a routine test but should be done only as indicated clinically.

10. Tests for Sexually Transmitted Diseases (STDs)

Men often have symptoms associated with many of the STDs, but this is not the case in all STD infections. Screening tests should include swabs of the genital area and penis as well as blood and urine tests. Those with more than one sexual partner or other high-risk behaviors such as drug use are at greatest risk for STDs.

11. Electrocardiogram (ECG)

An ECG can detect abnormalities in the heart, but it's only a single snapshot at a given moment in time. Don't kid yourself. It cannot detect all problems and is not as useful as a stress test in detecting underlying disease or blockages. It is worthwhile getting a baseline ECG around age thirty-five and then at other intervals as recommended by your physician.

12. Testicular Examination

Just as women should examine their breasts monthly, men should per-form monthly examinations on their testes beginning at adolescence. Testic-ular cancer is the most common malignancy in men in their early twenties and thirties. You should expect your doctor to perform a testicular exam as a part of every routine physical.

13. Fasting Blood Sugar Test

An FBS test measures the level of sugar or glucose in your blood after an eight-hour fast. It is a test for diabetes. You should be tested beginning at age forty and at the same intervals as cholesterol testing and CRP. If you are at risk for diabetes, are obese, have high blood pressure, are African-American, Native American, or Hispanic, you should be tested more frequently than groups not at risk. You should also be tested if you have the symptoms com-monly associated with diabetes, such as increased thirst, frequency of urina-tion, unexplained weight loss, and fatigue.

If you're already a diabetic, then at least twice a year or more, you should receive a test called the A1C. The A1C test measures the percentage of glu-cose attached to red blood cells in the bloodstream. If the A1C result is above 7 percent, the risk of illness from diabetes is greatly increased.

14. Eye Examination

Glaucoma (elevated pressure in the eye) is the most frequent cause of preventable blindness in the United States and is easily detectable during a good examination of the eyes. Such an exam can determine visual abnormal-ities that may require glasses. It can also determine the presence of cataracts (clouding of the lens of the eye) and macular degeneration (deterioration of cells in the back of the eye that affects us as we age). Prior to age fifty, an eye exam should be done every two to three years and more frequently after that.

Essential Medical Tests for Females

1. Blood Pressure Test

High blood pressure (or hypertension) is known as the "silent killer." Most of us have no symptoms when our blood pressure is high. The longer blood pressure goes undetected and untreated, the greater the risk of heart attack, stroke, heart failure, and kidney damage for both men and women. A blood pressure test should be done at least every two years when you're younger but annually over the age of forty. We're more conservative than many others when it comes to checking your pressure.

People with diabetes, who are overweight, or who have a family history of diabetes are at greatest risk for blood pressure problems and should be checked more frequently. African-Americans are more at risk for hypertension at earlier ages than whites, so they should be tested annually at a younger age.

Ideally, according to the latest guidelines we should try to keep our systolic (top number) below 120 and our diastolic (lower number) below 80 (see the new guidelines and classifications in Chapter 8). Hypertension begins at 140 systolic and 90 diastolic and should be treated, especially if a person is diabetic or has kidney disease.

2. Pap Smear *(see the chapter on cancer for more details)*

Pap tests are designed to detect precancerous and cancerous changes on a woman's cervix. Tests should begin at age eighteen or with the beginning of sexual activity—whichever comes first. If you have an abnormal result or you're sexually active with more than one person, an annual exam is recommended.

3. Colon Examination *(see the chapter on cancer for more details)*

Colorectal cancer is a cancer that is largely preventable with frequent exams. A fecal occult blood test is often used as a screening test, but by age fifty, a colonoscopy should be done. If your test results are normal, you don't have to be tested again for three to five years. If you're at higher risk for colon cancer because of family history, the test should be done at an earlier age and more frequently.

4. Clinical Breast Exam *(see the chapter on cancer for more details)*

Breast examination by a health care professional is key beginning at age eighteen. Your health care provider should teach you how to examine your own breasts at the time of the exam. These exams should take place every three years until age forty, when they should occur annually.

5. Mammogram *(see the chapter on cancer for more details)*

Follow the advice of your doctor and get these exams as directed. At the minimum, you should get one annually after age fifty.

6. Dental Examination

Although there are no firm guidelines from the CDC (Centers for Disease Control) on how often adults should get dental exams, for maximum oral health, you should see your dentist at least once a year for a comprehensive dental examination and at least twice a year for a cleaning of your teeth and gums. Many adults need to have periodontal (gum) cleanings more often than every six months—for many, once every three to four months is what is needed in order to keep your teeth and gums healthy and free of infection and disease.

Regular visits to the dentist can help:

- Prevent tooth decay.

- Prevent or treat gum disease (also known as periodontal disease).

- Prevent periodontal disease, which has been associated with increased risk of coronary artery disease and peripheral vascular disease, placing people at risk for heart attack or stroke.

- Prevent bacterial infections of the gums

At least, twice-yearly dental visits are especially important if you:

- Have diabetes, since poor control of insulin levels can result in gum disease.

- Smoke, since tobacco makes gum disease worse.

■ Take prescription or over-the-counter medications that reduce saliva (and make your mouth feel dry), placing individuals at risk for cavities and gum disease.

7. Bone Density Measurement

Women are at considerable risk for osteoporosis, a disease that causes loss of bone mass. Reduced bone mass increases the risk of fractures, even if you don't have a fall. Women sixty and older should be screened for osteoporosis using this test. Based on the test results your doctor will determine when you need to be retested. Based on your personal risk for osteoporosis, your doctor may give this test to you at an early age and more frequently.

8. Skin Examination

Skin cancer is the most common cancer in the United States, and those at greatest risk are those who have had the most sun exposure over the years. Most skin cancers can be removed before they cause further health problems. You should expect a complete skin examination at the time of your regular full physical examination. Skin exams should be performed regularly beginning at age forty because skin damage begins to show up later in life.

9. Cholesterol Tests *(see the chapter on cardiovascular disease for more details)*

You notice that we said tests and not a single test. Total cholesterol is an inadequate assessment of the impact of cholesterol on your arteries. Your doctor needs to measure HDL, LDL, and triglycerides as well. Only then can you know the risk you may have from cholesterol. Examinations should begin in your twenties and then take place every three to five years unless you have elevated levels of cholesterol.

10. C-Reactive Protein Test *(see the chapter on cardiovascular disease for more details)*

This is one of the newest tests that doctors are ordering and is a measure of inflammation in the body. Those with elevated levels of CRP are at increased risk for heart attacks and stroke. There are many different conditions that can elevate CRP and most are correctable. Tests should begin at age thirty and be repeated at the same time interval as cholesterol level testing.

11. Thyroid Stimulating Hormone (TSH) Test

TSH is a hormone made in the brain that stimulates the proper functioning of the thyroid. This test can detect whether or not your thyroid is producing too little or too much of the hormone thyroxine. Women need this test beginning at age thirty-five and then every five years unless they have a family history of thyroid problems or high cholesterol. If they do, they need the testing more often.

12. Urinalysis

Urine tests can detect the presence of infection. This is most important because women often can have urinary tract infections without symptoms, especially when they are pregnant. Red blood cells in the urine can signify a tumor or problems with your kidneys or bladder. Tests should take place during every routine complete examination or if symptoms suggest problems.

13. Complete Blood Count (CBC)

The CBC measures how well your bone marrow and immune system is working. It measures white blood cells (indicative of infection), hemoglobin and hematocrit (indicative of the ability of the blood to carry oxygen and the presence of anemia), and platelets (indicative of the clotting ability of the blood). It can help detect disorders of the blood. It is not a routine test but should be done only as indicated clinically.

14. Tests for Sexually Transmitted Diseases (STDs)

Women often have very few symptoms associated with many of the STDs, and if they do, these may not indicate the presence of infection. Screening tests should include swabs of the genital area, cervix, and urethra as well blood and urine tests. Those with more than one sexual partner or other high-risk behaviors such as drug use are at greatest risk for STDs.

15. Electrocardiogram (ECG)

An ECG can detect abnormalities in the heart, but it's only a single snapshot at a given moment in time. Don't kid yourself. It cannot detect all problems and is not as useful as a stress test in detecting underlying disease or blockages. It is worthwhile getting a baseline ECG around age thirty-five and then at other intervals as recommended by your physician.

16. Fasting Blood Sugar Test

An FBS test measures the level of sugar or glucose in your blood after an eight-hour fast. It is a test for diabetes. You should be tested beginning at age forty and at the same intervals as cholesterol testing and CRP. If you are at risk for diabetes, are obese, have high blood pressure, are African-American, Native American, or Hispanic, you should be tested more frequently than groups not at risk. You should also be tested if you have the symptoms commonly associated with diabetes, such as increased thirst, frequency of urination, unexplained weight loss, and fatigue.

If you're already a diabetic, then at least twice a year or more, you should receive a test called the A1C. The A1C test measures the percentage of glucose attached to red blood cells in the bloodstream. If the A1C result is above 7 percent, the risk of illness from diabetes is greatly increased.

17. Eye Examination

Glaucoma (elevated pressure in the eye) is the most frequent cause of preventable blindness in the U.S. and is easily detectable during a good examination of the eyes. Such an exam can determine visual abnormalities that may require glasses. It can also determine the presence of cataracts (clouding of the lens of the eye) and macular degeneration (deterioration of cells in the back of the eye that affects us as we age). Prior to age fifty, an eye exam should be done every two to three years and more frequently after that.

RISKS OF MEDICAL SCREENING OR TESTING

Doctors know that the more tests they order, the more likely they are to get a positive result (one outside the normal limits for that test). If you do twenty tests, there is a 5 percent chance that at least one test result will be outside of the normal range, but will turn out not to be abnormal when repeated or checked out further. This is known as a false positive test. Why does this occur? No matter how good, tests are not 100 percent accurate. Many are a lot less accurate than the ideal, and this is why some tests are not used or recommended as screening tests. If a test is only 80 percent accurate, it means that 20 percent of those tested over time could have false positive results. The more inaccurate a test, the more the person being tested is at risk. False positives can also occur because of improper administration of the tests, errors at the lab, and inaccurate readings of test results.

We can hear you saying, "What's the big deal about having a false positive test result? Why am I at risk?

False Positive Test Risks

The interventional cascade: When doctors get a positive test result, they just can't ignore it, but must pursue the results in an effort to confirm them. Some of the tests that are ordered to check out a positive test are not benign, and they can put a person at more risk for serious health problems. For instance, if someone has a positive cardiac stress test while on the treadmill, a physician might suggest a cardiac catheterization to determine the true extent of the problem. Unfortunately, false positives are very common in cardiac stress testing in both men and women. You decide to undergo the cardiac cath. This now puts you at a small risk of death and of serious cardiac arrhythmias or reactions to the dye that is used during the procedure. All because you had a false positive test in the first place. There was nothing really wrong with you, but your physician had to check out the abnormal result. This is a good example of what's known as the interventional cascade.

Labeling: You have a test result that's positive. If it is serious enough, you are now labeled with the results of that test and its clinical implications. Here's what we mean. As part of a routine physical, you have a complete blood test that checks out twenty-six different blood chemistry parameters in your blood. Two of these tests indicate slightly abnormal liver enzymes. These are not clinically significant abnormalities because you recently had a bout of infectious mononucleosis that caused these elevated liver enzymes, plus you just took an excess dose of acetaminophen (Tylenol) for a severe headache (this can also affect your liver tests for a few days). Despite these benign causes of abnormal liver tests, you are now labeled as having elevated liver enzymes. It may be enough to keep you from getting health insurance, life insurance, or maybe even certain jobs. It's not fair, but that's what happens.

Distrust of medical testing: Because of a bad experience with testing, patients may begin to mistrust medical testing and not go for routine testing or follow-up that they might need to prevent future health problems. Patients may not comply with what doctors ask because abnormal test results have engendered mistrust.

Severe patient anxiety: If you believe you have a certain disease, you change the way you act or live. What harm is done to a person when they believe they have some serious medical condition hanging over their heads? It's hard to estimate. If you are told that you have heart disease, some of you will likely worry because of every skipped beat or unexplained chest pain. A perfect example of this is how unethical lawyers scare people into believing they might have asbestos-related lung disease. They may advertise this deadly possibility and then a person gets a false-positive result. A radiologist overinterprets a chest X ray or CT scan of the lung and reports findings compatible with asbestosis. But in fact, the person has never had significant asbestos exposure; the abnormality on the scan may be due to smoking, natural aging, or some other cause. Now imagine the harm that's been done to the person who lives in fear of dying from cancer one day. It's unfair and unethical.

What happens if your doctor doesn't follow up on some abnormal test result you might have? If a medical problem develops as a result of a failure to diagnose it soon enough, it could be a case of malpractice because the doctor didn't aggressively pursue this abnormal test. So what do doctors do? They take the safe way out (and we can't blame them in most cases). They do whatever it takes to reassure the patient and themselves that the out-of-line results don't mean much. It costs you time and money.

WHY AREN'T WE GETTING SCREENED?

We'll bet that after you reviewed the list of tests that are important to your health, many of you realized that you haven't gotten some of them on a regular basis. At least that's been the case for most people we've surveyed. It's also borne out by a recent government study, which showed that more than half of all Americans do not receive many of the important preventive services they need. It's hard to believe since we're one of the richest countries on earth and we know that the tests we listed do prevent disease and do save money. Here are some of the reasons why most people don't get the preventive care they need:

- 44 million Americans have no health insurance, so they can't afford to get many of these services.

- Some people don't like to get some of the tests because they're embarrassed by what it takes to get the tests done—e.g., colon screening, Pap smears, testing stool for blood.

- People are confused over what tests are needed and when (hopefully, we've helped to remove this barrier).

■ Doctors aren't direct enough to their patients about getting preventive tests. Some managed care organizations don't encourage counseling on prevention, as it clearly has some up-front costs.

■ Employers and insurers have experienced double-digit increases in health care costs for the past few years. As a result, these plans are reducing or eliminating coverage in order to reduce costs. Preventive services and specialized testing are some of the things that are most frequently eliminated.

WHAT DOCTORS KNOW ABOUT
Medical Testing . . . And You Should Too

---

1. Preventive testing clearly identifies certain diseases before more severe complications occur. They can also reduce the chances of dying from specific diseases.

2. Doctors will not wait for their doctors to suggest preventive testing, but will be proactive in demanding tests when they are appropriate. They understand that it's a personal responsibility to get the care they need.

3. Just because a health plan chooses not to cover specific preventive testing that is recommended and considered worthwhile by many experts does not mean that the tests are not worthwhile. It may be worth paying for them outside such plans.

4. Doctors will appeal in writing any denials of coverage of preventive testing by insurers or employers. They will use the recommendations of medical organizations as the basis for this appeal. This puts the people who manage the insurance plan on notice and may cause them to change their policy on preventive testing.

5. Finding a doctor who is concerned about prevention of disease is an important factor in selecting a primary care doctor. If your doctor isn't concerned about prevention at many levels, then find another one who is.

WHY BOTHER YOUR DOCTOR? ORDER THE BLOOD TESTS YOU WANT ON-LINE

Direct-access blood testing may become one of the next big trends in medicine. How'd you like to be able to go down the street to your local medical laboratory and order blood tests without that long wait and hassle that often happens at your doctor's office? At first glance, it seems like a very nice idea, and believe it or not, you'll actually be able to get your results back in less than a week. Well, folks, the ability to order your own tests is here now, depending on where you live, and the trend is growing.

Qwest Diagnostics, a national commercial testing lab, has opened a number of sites that will allow medical consumers to choose from a menu of thirty to fifty tests. They even partnered with Giant Food, a grocery-store chain, to sell these tests in their stores. Here's how it works: You go to the lab, order your tests, pay with a credit card, and in most cases, get your results the next day off the Internet. It's quick, convenient, and much less of a hassle than going to most doctor's offices.

The Web-based outfits that offer these services do so by advertising on-line. The consumer picks the tests they want and then goes down to a local lab that the Web-based business has contracted with. The tests are then shipped out of state to be tested. The Web sites have some definite advantages over commercial labs because such direct-to-consumer businesses aren't prohibited from performing most blood tests without a doctor's authorization. Commercial labs aren't allowed to perform many tests unless a doctor orders them.

Direct-access testing is great for people who want to check their general health status, and for those who need regular periodic testing—diabetics, people with thyroid disease who are on medications, and those taking certain medications. Other people are using these tests to screen for diseases they want to keep confidential and to determine their health before switching health insurance or applying for life insurance (many companies will deny insurance if you have certain health problems).

Commercial labs do advise patients to see their doctor for follow-up once the tests are done, but there is no requirement that patients comply . . . and this is what concerns doctors. Many are afraid that patients will not follow up appropriately, especially if they get test results that they don't understand. They are worried that patients will fail to get the treatment they need. Another issue is that some patients will worry needlessly when a less important test is slightly abnormal. Our advice would be to always talk with your doctor about test results if you should decide to order them on your own. It could make a huge difference in your health.

TOTAL BODY SCAN: GOOD MONEY MAKER BUT BAD MEDICINE

Do you remember how fantastic it was in *Star Trek* when Dr. McCoy waved his magic scanner over someone's body and diagnosed some medical condition? It seemed so futuristic when we first viewed it. Who wouldn't want to avail themselves of such a marvel? Well, to a certain extent, this is now possible, thanks to a technology called the total body scan. The only problem is that it really makes no sense.

As we noted earlier in this chapter, we can perform multiple tests, but shotgun screening for rare diseases can be risky, expensive, and often inaccurate. Any diagnostic test produces a certain number of test results that are abnormal even though the patient is perfectly healthy (a false-positive result). Then the fun begins. More tests will be done in order to confirm these erroneous results. A cascade of tests now occurs. These additional tests can be risky and are almost always expensive.

Total body scans using CT scans or MRIs are a great example of a good idea gone bad . . . at least at this point in time. It capitalizes on the American misconception that more testing and more services equal more health. In 2002, there were over a hundred total body scanners in the United States, but experts estimate the number could reach four thousand by 2007. The persons most frequently targeted (and exploited, we might say) by vendors pushing body scans are corporate executives, who get these scans as part of "executive physical" programs. Vendors use the fear of cancer as one of their strong selling points for these scans. But not one reputable study has confirmed the benefits of total body scans. The cost for these exams is much more than any benefit gained by the rare executive who shows up with something.

However, one of the most appealing things about full body scans is how incredibly easy they are to get—with the promise of a big diagnosis in record time. Technicians attach three electrodes to you, then slide you through a big circular portal on a moving examination table (a little like a medical Disney ride), through a rotating X-ray tube. About a half a minute later, your torso has been scanned with 3-D digital images suitable for framing.

What do these scans show? Some proponents say they could benefit heart patients. When you get a full body scan, your heart is scanned and you are given a coronary score of zero to over 400. The higher the number, the higher the buildup of calcified plaque lining the walls of your arteries. In one study of 1,200 patients at St. Francis Hospital in Roslyn, New York, people with coronary scan scoring over 160 were thirty-five times more likely to have a heart attack within the next nineteen months than those with a score of zero. But you don't need a total body scan to learn such things; you could simply get a CT scan or MRI that focuses specifically on the arteries in your heart.

The best thing about these scans of your heart is that they are a great eye-opener. Seeing the plaque can jump-start you into a diet and exercise program. The thing to be careful of? If you have a low score, it doesn't mean that everything is fine. These scans do not measure for a lot of different heart-related problems; for example, plaque buildup that is soft, and not calcified, can be just as dangerous as calcified plaque, but is not measured by these scans. The scans also cannot detect prostate cancer, although this is certainly one condition that men would most want an instant test for.

Here's the bottom line: MRIs and CT scans need to be used as part of a testing program because your doctor suspects a problem, based on your particular medical situation. Our advice to you is that unless your doctor recommends one for your individual situation, you should avoid body scans and save yourself some money, avoid unneeded radiation, and eliminate the risk of further unneeded testing.

Summary

Preventive testing is essential for detecting disease before problems arise. Follow the recommended guidelines for your age and sex. Don't wait for your doctor to recommend these tests but take charge of your own health and insist on the tests that you need. After all, it's your health and your life.

CHAPTER FOUR

HOSPITALS: THEY CAN KILL YOU IF YOU'RE NOT CAREFUL

Would you knowingly double your risk of dying when you have a surgical procedure? Would you increase the chances of a loved one dying during a hospital stay? Of course not, but patients do these things all the time and don't even know it. Doctors know that the hospital they choose for surgery can often mean the difference between life and death. By making the right decision, you can increase your chance for a successful surgery and speedy recovery while cutting your risk of dying in half. When doctors go into the hospital, they know that where they are admitted is just as important as who is treating them.

In this chapter, we'll tell you how to choose your hospital if you have a choice (in emergency situations, this may not be possible); how to stay healthy in the hospital (believe it or not, you can get sicker just by being in one); and the best way to find the right hospital with the best surgical team for the surgery you need. The information in this chapter just might save your life.

WHAT DOCTORS KNOW ABOUT
Hospitals . . . And You Should Too

1. All hospitals are not equal when it comes to the type of services delivered.

2. The more surgeries of a certain type that a hospital does, the more successful the outcomes.

3. Specialized care units are vital for successful recovery.

4. In the case of a serious accident, go to a trauma center if at all possible. The more accident cases the trauma center handles, the better your chances for a successful outcome.

5. Doctors avoid hospitalization whenever possible.

6. Doctors take an active role in preventing medical errors and hospital-acquired infections.

NOT ALL HOSPITALS ARE CREATED EQUAL

Remember one thing, all hospitals can't be number one in the care they provide no matter what their advertisements may say. Some may provide better service, while others may excel at certain surgeries or medical treatments. Which hospital you choose should depend on what your medical problem is.

Different hospitals provide different levels of care, and you often can't tell just by looking at a hospital what that level of care is. In the most basic terms, hospitals are graded by the type and extent of the clinical services they deliver (primary, secondary, and tertiary level care).

A *primary care hospital* will deliver basic clinical services but will not have more advanced levels of care, nor will services be readily available twenty-four hours a day. (These are often rural hospitals or smaller specialty hospitals.) On the other hand, *a tertiary care hospital* has a complete range of clinical services, such as the ability to perform cardiac bypass surgery and provide complete trauma services. It also has all the necessary advanced support services—intensive care units, blood banks, and in-depth laboratory testing. (These are your referral hospitals that are found only in big cities.) In between these two levels of care are your *secondary hospitals.* They provide more expert care than a primary care hospital but not at the level of the tertiary care hospital.

We're going to use a simple analogy to illustrate these differences. If all you want to eat for dinner is a burger and fries, you're probably not going to eat at the most fancy or most expensive restaurant in town. If, however, you're craving beef Wellington, Yorkshire pudding, and a fancy dessert, only the expensive restaurant will have the more well-trained chef and the right equipment to prepare the meal you want. The same is true for hospitals. If all you need is your appendix out or a CT scan of your abdomen, a primary care hospital is perfect. If you need heart bypass surgery or you're a woman delivering a high-risk pregnancy, you need a tertiary care hospital.

Another point to consider when choosing a hospital: Do you prefer a teaching hospital or a nonteaching hospital? A teaching hospital is one that has a dean's committee and at least one residency program. This may mean that your private doctor is not the only one examining you and asking you questions. We feel that having other doctors or residents and students (doctors-in-training) ask you questions isn't a bad thing, plus you'll also be helping to educate the next generation of doctors. If you are going into the hospital for advanced surgery, you'll want to know whether or not there is a surgical teaching program. Just ask the hospital or your doctor and they can tell you the answer.

Several recent publications have found that the mortality (death) rate and the morbidity (complication) rates in teaching hospitals in urban settings are lower than those of nonteaching hospitals. The biggest reason for these differences may be that teaching hospitals have more up-to-date research and higher accountability processes available to support the teaching program. On the downside, some experts have found that when resident physicians are the primary surgeons on some operations, they often have a slightly higher complication rate in surgery.

Even with this apparent trade-off, and everything else being equal, if a doctor were a patient, he or she would still more likely choose a teaching hospital over a nonteaching facility. You can always ask that a resident not be the primary surgeon on your case. You always have the right to ask this and you should always be told who the primary physician performing your operation will be when you sign your consent form.

FINDING THE BEST HOSPITAL

One way to judge a hospital is to find out where the top doctors in an area put their patients. You can get the names of the top doctors from local medical support groups; they often know who the top docs are. You can also use magazine surveys of top doctors. These articles do miss many excellent doctors who haven't been in practice as long, or might not have published as many articles, but they give you a good idea of who some of the best doctors are. A hospital where the top doctors practice is usually a very good hospital, and one doctors would choose if they needed care.

Hospitals are also graded. The Internet is one of the best sources for information about an easy-to-understand grading system for hospitals across the United States. It's a Colorado-based health care company called HealthGrades and it can be found at www.healthgrades.com. It's the only consumer-oriented source for data on five thousand hospitals nationwide and for many of the surgical and hospital procedures they perform.

HealthGrades rates hospitals using a five-star (best), three-star (acceptable), and one-star (poorest) rating system based on Medicare data. Using a proprietary formula, it further ranks the hospitals in performing various high-risk surgical and other invasive procedures like bypass surgery, heart attacks, hip and knee replacements, and angioplasty. It even provides data on death rates and complication rates. And all the information is available free of charge when you go to their Web site.

You'll be able to answer such questions as: "How does this particular hospital rank in comparison to others for a particular surgical procedure?" "What rate of serious complications did patients have who underwent a particular surgery at a specific hospital and how does this compare to other hospitals?" "How often did patients die who had a particular surgical procedure at a hospital?" These are the questions that anyone undergoing surgery or serious hospital procedures should ask, and HealthGrades is the only national Web site that can help you to answer them at this moment.

HealthGrades data is released each year, usually in the fourth quarter. Here's some information comparing five-star hospitals to one-star hospitals culled from HealthGrades' most recent report.

- Cardiac bypass surgery: The death rate is three times higher at one-star hospitals than at five-star hospitals.

- Heart attack: The death rate is two times higher at one-star hospitals than at five-star hospitals.

- Stroke: One-star hospitals have a death rate from strokes three times higher than five-star hospitals.

- Aortic aneurysm: The death rate is five times higher as one-star hospitals than at five-star hospitals.

Even though five-star hospitals often have sicker patients, people often fare better at these facilities.

To put these findings into perspective: If the patients included in this study had gone to a five-star hospital over a one-star hospital, potentially almost twenty-five thousand lives might have been saved during the last three years. It's clear from this year's data that making an informed choice can be a matter of life and death.

A couple of states, New York and California, have published some additional data about surgeries and procedures at local facilities. Otherwise, most other rankings of hospitals consider financial data and operational data along with hospital outcome data in their computations. We don't think they're as good to use.

Internet Information Sites for Hospitals

www.healthgrades.com: HealthGrades is a Colorado-based company providing the only consume-oriented objective "report card" ratings on hospitals and health care providers nationwide. This group ranks five thousand hospitals all across the country using a proprietary formula based on many factors, and provides ratings on cardiac bypass surgery, hip replacements, vascular surgery, pulmonary medicine, and cardiology. You can also find information on nursing homes, assisted living centers, home health agencies, and fertility clinics.

www.healthscope.org: The Pacific Business Group on Health, a nonprofit coalition of businesses, sponsors this site and includes information on most Southern California hospitals. It provides data on a wide variety of surgical procedures and high-risk conditions, as well as death rates. It contains information on C-section rates, angioplasty, heart attack survival rates, coronary bypass rates, and survival rates of premature babies to mention a few.

www.healthcarechoices.org: Health Care Choices is a nonprofit consumer group based in New York City that posts surgical volume information for many procedures on its Web site. It gets information from available databases and allows patients to do multistate searches to find quality hospitals within a reasonable distance.

Report cards are useful in promoting informed decision-making in patients, but only if patients/consumers begin to use them. In one study, only 12 percent of patients in Pennsylvania utilized statewide report cards on cardiac surgery and less than 1 percent knew the correct rating of their heart surgeon or hospital. Doesn't say much for our willingness to use these useful tools. Patients have to take responsibility to educate themselves.

When report card information is provided to policy makers, surgeons, and hospitals, even if confidential, improvements in death rates after cardiac bypass surgery have been noted in many instances. It's been proven in Canada, New York, Pennsylvania, and Massachusetts, to mention a few.

Finding the Right Hospital for Your Surgery: The Higher Surgical Volume, the Lower the Risk

Surgery, no matter how minor, is not something to be undertaken lightly. A myriad of complications can occur. All nonsurgical treatment options should be explored and the benefits of surgery must outweigh any potential risks. In the next chapter, we'll give you guidelines for determining when surgery is the best option and choosing the right surgeon. For now, let's focus on finding the right hospital if you do have to go in for a surgical procedure.

Practice makes perfect, or the more often you do something, the better you usually become at it. These very simple axioms hold true for medicine as well as many other things in life. Do you remember the first time you rode a bike or drove a car? You probably weren't very good at it, but with practice, your skill level improved dramatically and your risk of accidents declined. This is true with hospitals as well. They generally become better at performing a particular surgery the more they do it.

In the April 2002 issue of the *New England Journal of Medicine*, a team of researchers reported their findings on the relationship between the number of specific cardiac and cancer surgeries performed at particular hospitals and the chances of a person dying (the mortality rate). They made the following statement about high-volume hospitals (those who perform a large number of specific high-risk surgeries): "In the absence of other information about the quality of surgery at the hospitals near them, Medicare patients undergoing selected cardiovascular or cancer procedures can significantly reduce their risk of operative death by selecting a high-volume hospital."

In other words, if you don't have any idea how to judge the quality of surgery at a hospital, the more high-risk heart or cancer surgeries a hospital does, the better they usually are at it. This wasn't the first time that this relationship between volume and outcome had been identified. A similar study published in the *Journal of the American Medical Association (JAMA)* identified eleven high-risk surgical procedures for which hospital experience is critical. The results were equally shocking and dramatic. The study showed that:

- in the case of surgical repair of an abdominal aortic aneurysm (a ballooning artery in the belly), hospitals doing fewer procedures had almost two-thirds more people die than did those hospitals doing more cases

- heart transplant patients are twice as likely to die at centers doing eight or fewer transplants than at centers doing more

- low-volume centers performing pediatric heart surgery had a 42 percent higher death rate than high-volume centers

The same relationship is true for surgeries on the arteries leading to the brain (carotid endarterectomies). The more of these procedures that a hospital and surgeon does, the better the results for the patients.

In 1998, the *American Journal of Public Health* published a study that showed that the odds of living five years after breast cancer surgery were less than half as good for women whose surgery was done in hospitals that performed 10 or fewer surgeries per year than for women who chose hospitals that performed 150 or more. Similar long-term benefits also seem to result when having ovarian, pancreatic, or rectal surgery at high-volume hospitals.

The risk of dying is clearly related to the number of specific complex surgical procedures done at a particular hospital. The Leapfrog Group, a coalition of more than eighty large public and private purchasers insuring about 25 million people, believes that the volume of surgeries at a hospital is so critical to the ultimate success of a surgery that they have set minimum volume numbers for specific surgeries to help reduce risk. The system is not perfect, and the specific numbers could be argued, but it's a good starting point for judging quality. The Leapfrog Group states that the following are the minimum number of surgeries to be done per year to lower the risk of dying:

Coronary bypass:	500
Angioplasty:	400
Carotid endarterectomy:	100
Pediatric heart surgery:	100
Prostate surgery:	55
Mastectomy:	25
Repair of abdominal aortic aneurysm:	30
Pancreatic cancer surgery:	10
Heart transplant:	9

Obviously these are just guidelines and don't take into consideration the skill of certain surgeons and the ability of certain smaller-volume hospitals to provide excellent care. But in the absence of other data, it's something to strongly consider.

In less complex surgical procedures, the relationship between number of surgeries and mortality/morbidity does not seem to be present. There appears to be no difference between low-volume and high-volume hospitals in less complex surgeries like simple hip fractures and cholecystectomies (removal of the gallbladder). This is not to say that patients can't die or have very serious problems as a result of the surgery, but the inherent risk is lower and the supporting team does not have to be as skilled.

So, which hospital should you choose? It's a no-brainer as far as we're concerned. In the absence of other information, we'd always choose a high-volume hospital.

Now, hospitals often don't report their surgical statistics, their rates of complications, or their death statistics to the public. They often give the excuse that the public really won't understand the numbers unless they are put into context. The hospitals are concerned about potential litigation, and they don't want to be compared without careful consideration of the severity of the underlying illness that a patient might bring to the surgery. The sicker the patient, the more likely they are to die or have serious operative complications. However, doctors demand to know these statistics before they go into surgery. Doctors take these statistics very seriously when they need an operation and that's why you should too.

It can't be any clearer. If you want to increase your chances of survival, pick a hospital that has performed the surgery you need many times. The more they do, the better they get, and the lower your risk.

INTENSIVE CARE UNITS: SPECIALIZED STAFFING SAVES LIVES

Congratulations! You've made it to the hospital safely after your heart attack, or you've just made it out of surgery successfully. In most hospitals (except smaller ones), you'd now be sent to one of your hospital's intensive care units: with a heart attack, you'd be placed in the CCU (coronary care unit); with a stroke, you'd be in the Medical ICU (intensive care unit); and after surgery, you'd be transferred to the surgical ICU. Intensive care units are where the sickest, most critical patients are put until they are functioning well enough to be cared for on a regular hospital ward.

Studies clearly show that patients who have the same severity of illness die less often and have fewer complications when cared for by expert physicians trained in critical care. These specialized doctors are called intensivists and their care has dramatically improved the survival rates in ICUs. If your hospital utilizes full-time specially trained physicians to staff its intensive care units, your risk of complications and death is reduced by as much as 30 percent. The use of intensivists, researchers estimate, can save as many as 150,000 lives annually. The problem is that only about 10 percent of hospitals employ full-time intensivists. Why? Part of the reason is cost. ICUs require specially trained physicians, nurses, and support staff—and they cost money. Intensive care units are among the costliest units in any hospital and carry the highest cost per patient per day. It all comes down to the bottom line.

Another reason for less than fully staffed ICUs is a tremendous shortage of these specialists. To try to meet this shortage of intensivists, some hospitals are turning to high-tech monitoring equipment. One company, Visicu, has developed a system called "eICU" to electronically monitor several hospital ICUs at one time. Hospitals in the Sentara health system in Virginia have already saved hundreds of lives using this system. One person compared eICU to an air-traffic controller monitoring a number of planes at one time and then stepping in if there's trouble.

How do you know how your hospital staffs its ICUs? The easiest way to know is to ask your hospital whether or not they employ intensivists full-time. You can also check a couple of Web sites for information.

www.leapfroggroup.org: The Leapfrog Group is an employer health care coalition group that focuses on quality-of-care issues. It provides a great deal of information on hospitals and intensive care units that meet its standards.

www.icu-usa.com: This Web site contains information about getting the best care in hospital intensive care units.

Here's some inside information that you need to know. There are two kinds of models for ICU's: an *open unit,* where private attending physicians contribute to and control the care of their patients; and a *closed unit,* where only specially trained intensivists provide for patients' medical needs. This day-to-day, hour-to-hour focus by intensive care physicians seems to be the most important reason for the reduced death rates and complication rates. Our recommendation: If you're having serious surgery or have a serious medical problem, and you have a choice of hospitals, choose the hospital that has full-time trained critical care specialists (intensivists) on staff. It will clearly increase your odds of living when you are very seriously ill.

TRAUMA CENTER AS AN OPTION

Doctors know that the best outcomes for trauma patients occur when patients go to dedicated trauma centers. The belief is that higher patient volume will lead to greater experience in caring for persons with severe trauma, and this experience will translate into better ultimate outcomes for patients. The data supports this assumption. There is strong evidence indicating that severely injured trauma patients with the highest risk of problems have a lesser chance of dying and are more likely to get out of the hospital sooner when they are treated at major trauma centers that handle in excess of 650 cases per year. It's clear that the experience of both the surgeons and the hospital support staff does make a difference. If you or your loved ones are seriously hurt, have the ambulance crew or helicopter team take you to the nearest trauma center.

WHAT DOCTORS KNOW ABOUT
Surgery . . . And You Should Too

The choice is clearly ours. You can help reduce the risk of dying in surgery by carefully selecting where you go for surgery and who performs your surgery, and by paying attention to the number of times any given facility has done that particular procedure. Here are some things that you can do to improve your chances for a better outcome:

1. When given a choice, choose a teaching hospital over a nonteaching hospital when all other things are equal. The teaching hospital will often have more of the support services that you need.

2. Request volume information and death rate data from the surgeon and the hospital where the surgery is to be done if it is a high-risk procedure.

3. If your surgeon or hospital hassles you about providing the volume or mortality information, or doesn't have such information, go find yourself another surgeon or hospital.

4. Get on the Internet and access information about hospitals from respected sources.

5. If surgical volume is low and the death rate high at the hospital you're considering, go elsewhere.

6. If a family member has a major accident, get them to a trauma center for care as soon as possible, as your chances of success are better . . . even if it means transferring them when they are stable.

HOSPITALS . . . HOW TO GET BACK OUT SAFELY

Sometimes, no matter what we do, or how hard we try to keep ourselves healthy, we have to be admitted to the hospital for surgery or for treatment of an illness or medical problem. Hospitals generally do a wonderful job caring for people, but despite the best intentions of those delivering care, you can actually become sicker just by being in the hospital. Doctors know this and try to avoid hospitalization whenever possible. Hospital-acquired infections, lack of care due to nursing shortages, medication errors, and inexperience in caring for certain conditions lead the list of reasons why bad things can happen to good people. This section is about taking steps to ensure that your hospital stay is as safe as possible.

HOSPITALS CAN KILL YOU, SO BE CAREFUL

In 1999, the Institute of Medicine (IOM) issued a report entitled *To Err Is Human.* Its central point was indisputable: Too many patients are suffering severe consequences that could, and should, be avoided. The IOM estimated that between 44,000 and 98,000 patients die each year as a result of preventable mistakes made in hospitals. These mistakes include medication mix-ups, faulty diagnoses, wrong surgeries, and hospital acquired infections because doctors and hospital staff didn't do something as simple as washing their hands. Total national costs (lost income, lost household production, and disability and health care costs) of preventable adverse events (medical errors resulting in injury of some kind) are estimated to be between $17 billion and $29 billion, of which health care costs represent over one-half.

The shocking part of all these numbers is that some experts believe that the IOM report likely *under*estimates the extent of preventable medical injuries for a few important reasons. First, the conclusions are based solely on data extracted from medical records and most injuries and most errors are not recorded in the medical record. Second, the IOM estimates are low because they don't include outpatient injuries or errors. There is no reason to believe that the percentage of errors should be any lower in this setting. Finally, in-depth studies reveal even higher rates of problems than those claimed in the IOM report—20 percent of deaths from heart attacks, pneumonia, and strokes were preventable, and 64 percent of in-hospital cardiac arrests were preventable. Do we have your attention yet?

> The IOM estimated that between 44,000 and 98,000 patients die each year as a result of preventable mistakes made in hospitals.

We may have gotten your attention,

but the previous report has not gotten the attention of those charged with educating medical students and residents on the subject. A recent research letter in the *Journal of the American Medical Association* (September 2001) reported that only 16 percent of all internal medicine clerkships in the survey had formal lectures on adverse drug reactions/interactions. Sadly, 35 percent of clerkship directors had little or no familiarity with the IOM's report on medical errors and how to reduce them. Medicine still has a long way to go in improving the care that is delivered. It's hard to argue with these statistics, isn't it?

NOSOCOMIAL INFECTIONS AND ANTIBIOTIC RESISTANCE

Each year some 2 million patients get infections while in a health care facility, and nearly ninety thousand will die as a result. How does this happen? Some patients will acquire an in-hospital infection that is transmitted by an unclean instrument, or a health care provider who didn't do all they could to keep a wound sterile, or maybe it was just being in contact with another sick patient. These hospital-acquired infections are called *nosocomial infections,* and they can often be more severe because the bacteria found in hospitals are more resistant to many antibiotics and because you as a patient may not be at your healthiest.

Centers for Disease Control (CDC) officials estimate that a full 70 percent of the bacteria that cause hospital-acquired infections are resistant to the most commonly used antibiotics. This makes these infections much more difficult to treat and extremely costly. The most alarming

> Each year some 2 million patients get infections while in a health care facility, and nearly ninety thousand will die as a result.

concern is that one day in the very near future we won't have any antibiotics left to fight these resistant bacteria.

Hospitals have just recently begun to collect and share this information. Prior to this, the concern was that the data could be leaked, and cause all sorts of lawsuits and financial problems for hospitals. Fortunately, the benefits of gathering more information outweighed these concerns: without data, no one knows where the problems lie and what can be done to reduce the likelihood of hospital acquired infections.

Believe it or not, the most common cause of nosocomial or hospital acquired infections is improper hand-washing hygiene among health care workers. Most studies show that compliance with guidelines for proper hand hygiene is less than 50 percent in hospitals. And who do you think the worst offenders are? We hate to say it, but doctors are far worse than nurses when it comes to washing their hands as they should.

The average person carries between ten thousand and 10 million bacteria on each hand. So, in order to reduce the risk of spreading infections from patient to patient, health care professionals should wash their hands before they see a patient in the hospital (it applies equally to the medical office setting). This is such a monumental problem in hospitals that the Centers for Disease Control have just issued new guidelines that urge doctors and nurses to abandon soap and water and begin using new fast-drying alcohol gels. Not only do the alcohol gels kill more bacteria and viruses, but they are also quicker and easier to use. It should take a full minute to wash with soap and water and it requires a sink and running water. The alcohol gels can be carried in a little vial, requires no special equipment, and dries in seconds. (This gel can be found in supermarkets and is great for using around the house or when anywhere from home.)

So why are we telling you all this? Because we want you to hold your health care provider's feet (really hands) to the fire, so to speak. We want you to realize the importance of hand washing in the prevention of hospital-acquired infections. Doctors know to ask their nurse or doctor if they've washed their hands before touching them or before changing a dressing or an IV line going into their body. Why take a chance? It takes only a few seconds to prevent an infection that could cause a lifetime of misery.

The CDC knows that this is such a problem that it's begun a National Nosocomial Infection Surveillance System to help hospitals conduct voluntary infection monitoring. Only about 315 hospitals participate in this program now, but infections in intensive care units have dropped 44 percent in hospitals that provide data. Community leaders should be asking hospitals why they aren't participating in this voluntary CDC effort. How can any hospital justify people going into their hospital and getting sicker instead of better?

Some hospital systems have taken an aggressive approach to solving hospital-acquired infections. The Pittsburgh Regional Healthcare Initiative is a coalition of health care providers, employers, insurers, corporations, and employees formed to improve health care delivery in the area. This group has set a goal to completely eliminate hospital-acquired infections and medication errors among its forty hospitals. It's an ambitious goal that can only help the people served by the group. What's your hospital doing to combat this very serious problem? It might be good to find out before you put yourself at risk.

WHERE HAVE ALL THE NURSES GONE?

Remember seeing how nurses were depicted in some of the old TV shows like *Dr. Kildare* or *St. Elsewhere*? They actually interacted with patients. They took blood pressures, spoke to patients, and knew them better than anyone else on the hospital staff did—even better than some doctors. You can still see this today with nurses in the intensive care units and emergency departments, but for many nurses, their jobs have changed dramatically. They do have some interactions with patients, but many are now forced to spend much of their time on administrative duties and paperwork. Because of these other job demands, less skilled and less well-trained hospital personnel are now doing some of the nursing duties previously performed by RNs. Registered nurses also have less time with patients because there are now fewer nurses available to work, thanks to a nationwide nursing shortage.

Unrealistic workloads are causing nurses to leave the profession in alarming numbers. Twenty percent of nurses in one study indicated that they were going to leave their current jobs within a year. Burnout among nurses exceeds other health care workers by 40 percent, while job dissatisfaction far exceeds the average for all U.S. workers. The problem is so bad in California that legislators have passed a law reducing patient-to-nurse ratios in hopes of reducing the nurse shortage.

A quarter of all hospital deaths or injuries to patients has been attributed to the nationwide nursing shortage. In a 2002 report, the Joint Commission on Accreditation of Healthcare Organizations called the nursing shortage "a prescription for danger." Patients have a greater chance of dying after surgery in hospitals where nurses have to take care of more patients. A study in the *Journal of the American Medical Association* in 2002 noted that having nurses care for six patients rather than four translated into a 14 percent increase in death; in the case of those with eight patients versus four the death rate increased to almost 31 percent. Tell me these statistics don't scare you a bit.

Because there are fewer nurses available to fill skilled nursing slots in hospitals, other nurses are forced to work longer hours and be responsible for more patients, and thus they have less time for overseeing less skilled support staff. All of these factors contribute to the increased errors in the hospital and a decreased amount of time with patients to monitor their medical conditions. Often it was the nurse who alerted the physician that there was a problem with his or her patient. Without this early warning system, patients' conditions may deteriorate and go undetected until it's too late.

So, what should each of us be doing about this? We can urge our local hospitals to hire more nurses at a wage that will attract and retain these health care professionals. If you are in the hospital, ask your nurse how many patients she has to care for on a given day. The more patients she or he has, the more cautious we urge you to be about ensuring that the right medicines are being given and the right follow-up care is taking place.

Christine's Comments

When my grandmother was hospitalized when her lung collapsed, I was able to confirm something that I always believed to be important: If at all possible, there should be a family member, a friend, or if that's not possible and if your resources allow, a private nurse, with you 24/7 during any hospital stay that you might have to face.

My grandmother, because of the pain medication that she was on and due to her advanced age, was too weak and too sedated to be able to get the nursing staff's attention when she was uncomfortable, hungry, or needed something. And the nurses caring for her, although extremely competent, were just too busy to constantly check in on her. But because someone from my family was always with (we took turns staying with her in rotations, around the clock), we were able to be her voice for her. We were able to get the doctors and the nurses who were on staff to get her what she needed—when she needed it.

Because often there are too few nurses charged with caring for too many patients. I strongly suggest that friends, family members or a private nurse stay in the hospital with patients who are seriously ill, elderly or young children. Most nurses will gladly assist a patient, but it helps to have someone to get the nurses attention and get what the patient needs.

DOCTOR'S OFFICES AND MEDICAL ERRORS

The Institute of Medicine's report focuses on hospital errors, but the great majority of patient visits occur in an outpatient setting—in doctor's offices. Outpatient care is more complex and less regulated than inpatient hospital care, so the risk of errors may be substantially higher.

In 2002, the *Family Practice Management* journal reported some of the results of a look at medical errors found by a group of family physicians in their practices. These errors were serious enough that the doctors stated that they didn't want them to happen again. Gaps in "knowledge and skills" accounted for only a minority of errors. More than 80 percent came from administrative or system errors. This means lapses in patient follow-up, misfiling or never documenting receipt of laboratory work, and miscommunication among hospitals, physicians, and patients.

What does this mean for you or your family member? It could mean that your physician never saw the report from the radiologist explaining a small lump on your mammogram, so the results were never communicated to you until it was too late. It could mean that the your gynecologist's recommendation of a repeat Pap smear was missed. It could mean that the letter from the cardiologist suggesting a medication change for his or her patient with heart failure was overlooked, and maybe that change would have been enough to prevent heart failure in the future.

Let's use a very practical example of why the best physicians have systems in place to help them care for their patients. Some people require the medication coumadin or warfarin to help prevent clotting. A person on coumadin requires very close monitoring to ensure the proper dose because doses vary as widely from one person to another. Failure to monitor closely can cause either life-threatening bleeding or an inability to prevent clotting. Patients on coumadin must have regular blood tests to monitor the medicine. Unbelievably, many physicians are saying to patients, "If you don't hear from us in a couple of days, give us a call and we'll let you know how to adjust your medicine." This makes the patient responsible for follow-up. We believe this is totally unacceptable. Follow-up needs to occur immediately and not in couple of days. If the dose is too high, the risk of bleeding complications is present for a couple of days. If too low, clotting may not be adequately prevented. Wouldn't you prefer the physician's office to have a system in place that alerts them that results should be back and the patient needs to be called? I know we would, and doctors would too. Look for a practice that has these types of systems in place. It can only reduce the chance for medical errors and help you in the long run.

Another major problem noted in the *FPM* journal was a lack of coordination between physician offices and emergency departments, skilled nursing facilities, and home health care services. Almost half of reported errors regarding coordination of services were associated with adverse consequences, including hospital admission and death. What are the implications for you and your family? You should double-check that your physician's office is aware of test results, has called in medications to nursing homes when they said they would, or has gotten results of tests done in an emergency room. Here's an example of what can go wrong:

A close friend of ours developed abdominal pain while on a business trip in another city. He decided to go to an emergency room to get help. He was kept overnight and had numerous tests done, including a CT scan of the abdomen. He began feeling better, so he left the hospital the next morning and returned home immediately. He called his doctor's office and told them of his visit to the ER. They said that they'd follow up with the ER and call him back if more testing had to be done. The doctor's office never called, and one day later our friend was brought to his local ER with severe abdominal pain. His appendix had ruptured and he also happened to have a kidney stone. Both of these things were on his CT scan at the other hospital but were missed by the ER doctor, so they were not seen until the radiologist read the film late on the day after the patient left the hospital. Because his doctor's office never called the ER, they didn't get the radiologist's report faxed to them. If they had gotten it, maybe an acute admission could have been avoided.

Need we say more? In our example, both the original hospital and our friend's doctor's office could have done better. It's too easy for things to fall through the cracks if systems and processes aren't in place to catch such things, especially when the hospital or office is extremely busy.

REDUCING MEDICAL ERRORS: DOESN'T ANYONE CARE?

So, what can be done to reduce medical errors? Patient safety can immediately be improved through better physician-patient communication. One of the root causes for medical errors in physician offices as well as in hospital is poor patient-physician communication. The Agency for Healthcare Research and Quality (AHRQ) found that physicians aren't doing enough to help their patients make informed decisions. Patients who are uninvolved and uninformed are less likely to follow their doctors' recommendations and comply with suggested treatments. Patients who don't feel comfortable talking with their doctors are less likely to ask questions that concern them or share information that it is needed by the doctor to make the best care decisions. A patient may not reveal that they are using over-the-counter medicines or herbal supplements that can interfere with prescribed medications. A physician may forget to specifically ask about the use of such drugs. Patient-physician communication is the core of the problem.

The bottom line: The responsibility for preventing medical errors rests with physicians and patients. The AHRQ has compiled a twenty-tip fact sheet to help prevent medical errors. The list helps patients to think outside the box and urges them *not* to assume that every health professional involved in their care knows everything he or she needs to know about their medical history. The AHRQ fact sheet can be obtained by calling 1-800-358-9295 or can be downloaded from the AHRQ Web site at <u>www.ahrq.gov/consumer.pathqpack.htm</u> (we have included many of these tips in this book).

Why don't we hear more about the problem of medical errors? It's hard to believe, but there hasn't been a champion who's come forward to move the health care system into action to make the needed changes. Surprisingly, consumers are silent on this issue. The media only reports anecdotal cases of problems. Hospital accrediting and licensing organizations only touch on the problem of medical errors peripherally when performing their inspections, and even these minimal efforts are met with resistance because of the increased costs associated with fixing the problem. Providers are leery of systematically uncovering and learning from errors because of the fear of being hauled into court.

Finally, a couple of the biggest obstacles to needed reform are employers and group purchasers of health insurance. Very few are truly concerned about quality of care or safety but are focused only on one thing—cost.

Likewise, most third party payment systems provide almost no reimbursement incentives for health care organizations to improve the safety or the quality of care. It's sad but true. For them, it's all about the bottom line. They have data to show what physicians deliver the best care, but it's easier for these insurance companies and managed care organizations to lump physicians into a single fee structure. It's not fair, but this is what's done in most cases today.

So, what's the answer? Consumer groups with huge clout like the American Association of Retired Persons (AARP) and professional physician organizations need to make safety and quality-of-care issues priorities on their agendas. There is no excuse for so many preventable deaths in our system of health care.

The problem of medical error is not fundamentally due to lack of medical knowledge. Simple measures of known effectiveness, such as unit dosing, marking the correct side of the body before surgery, twenty-four-hour availability of pharmacists and emergency physicians, are often ignored. Health care refuses to learn what industries like the airlines have already learned: Safe performance cannot be expected from workers who are sleep deprived, who work double or triple shifts, or whose job involves multiple or competing urgent priorities.

Another factor contributing to medical errors, and especially to adverse drug events, is the lack of complete information on a patient. When patients see multiple providers in different settings, none of whom have all the required medical information, it's easy for something to go wrong.

Drug interactions are obviously an extremely serious problem with tremendous impact on the health and finances of this country, not to mention on the people who suffer them. Some of the symptoms of drug interactions include confusion, falling, weight loss, dizziness, and changes in behavior or moods.

So what can you do to reduce your chances of getting a hospital-acquired infection or having a hospital error cause problems for you?

Ten Ways to Reduce Hospital Errors and Infections

1. Choose a hospital at which many patients have had the procedure or surgery that you need.

Kevin's Comments

While in the ER, I used to see patients who didn't know what medicines they were taking, what their actual diagnoses were, and what their test results really showed. I felt like a pilot flying blind. In most cases I had no way to get their medical records, so I had to guess at the best course of treatment or the best drugs to give them. Without that information, I could have given a medication that interacted with a drug they were already taking and caused even further problems.

I can't tell you how many times I would ask patients in the ER what medicines they were currently taking so that I could safely write what was needed that night or see if their current meds could be causing some of their symptoms. Most of the time, patients did not know exactly what they were taking or in what dosage. I heard time and time again, "I'm not exactly sure what I'm taking, but I think it's for high blood pressure and it's a little blue pill." That kind of information didn't help me a bit. It just increased the chances for a potentially serious drug interaction.

2. Make sure all your doctors agree on what will be done while in hospital.

3. When in the hospital, make sure that all hospital workers that come in contact with you have washed their hands.

4. Always keep a list of the medications you're on and the dosage in your wallet.

5. Whenever you are given a medicine in the hospital, ask what it is and why it's being given to you.

6. Ask a friend or family member to be there as your advocate and to record things so you don't forget.

7. Ask why a test is being done and how it will change your treatment.

8. Learn as much as you can about your condition from reliable sources.

9. Make sure that your hospital has a reporting system for hospital-acquired infections and has an aggressive infection control plan. If not, go elsewhere for your care.

10. When being discharged, have your doctor explain what the exact treatment plan at home should be and write it down.

Summary

Reducing medical errors is a problem for all of us. You can't be passive but have to be actively engaged in your care and treatment. An informed, engaged patient is the best help for your doctor. Get involved locally with your health care provider and work toward implementing systems to reduce medical errors and adverse events. Believe it or not, you, and your family or supporting friends, can make a difference.

CHAPTER FIVE

SURGERY: TO CUT OR NOT TO CUT IS THE QUESTION

If you question a surgeon, he or she will always tell you that no operation, no matter how simple, is always the same. Things can and do go wrong in something as simple as an appendectomy. No surgery is without risk, despite the best intentions of everyone involved. Surgeons have operated on the wrong leg of patients. Wrong medications have been given during surgery or after surgery. Surgeons have performed an operation they didn't have the skills to do. It's disturbing and alarming to hear these things, but it's a fact of life.

In this chapter, we'll teach you some of the key questions to ask if one of your doctors recommends surgery. Don't think that it can't happen to you. Thirty-five million Americans undergo operations every year. But a good many of them may not be necessary. We'll help you explore some of the things you can do to protect yourself or a family member and improve your odds for success if you're ever told that surgery is needed.

Let's first look at a hypothetical situation:

You've had low back pain for weeks and it seems to be getting worse. You see your family doctor who refers you to an orthopedic surgeon for further evaluation. After a brief exam by the surgeon, you're told that you need surgery. Despite the many questions you have going through your mind, you decide that he or she wouldn't have recommended surgery if it hadn't been in your best interest. So, you immediately schedule surgery for the very near future.

Change the type of surgery and the specialty of the surgeon and you have a typical scene that's repeated in doctors' offices all across the country every day. So, what's wrong with this picture? In many cases, there may be nothing wrong with it. But patients do need to be less passively trusting, and need to know that they often may have other options. If a doctor or his or her family member were the patient in the above scenario, we doubt that it would have gone exactly the same way.

What would a doctor do? Let us assure you that prior to any surgery, a doctor would have immediately asked a great many questions. In this chapter, we'll teach you what the most important questions are. In the example above, we would hope you'd ask some of the following:

- Is an orthopedic surgeon the best choice, or is a neurosurgeon the better choice?

- Are there other alternatives that should be used prior to referral to a surgeon, i.e. medicines or physical therapy?

- Should more definitive testing be done prior to the referral to better define the problem?

- What can I expect from surgery and what questions should I be sure to ask my surgeon?

- Are you referring me to the doctor you would use?

These are just a few of the questions your doctor would know to ask . . . and that you should be asking before scheduling any surgery.

WHAT DOCTORS KNOW ABOUT
Surgery . . . And You Should Too

1. Surgery is not without risks, no matter how minor it is. Ask about the risks and look for alternatives when you can.

2. Not all surgeons are created equal. Be very careful about the surgeon you pick.

3. A general surgeon is not the best surgeon for most high-risk procedures.

4. Be just as cautious when choosing the hospital you go to and your anesthesia team.

5. There are things you can do to reduce the risk of problems before and after surgery.

6. Once the actual surgery is complete, the real healing begins. Rehabilitative care or physical therapy should often be an essential part of that surgical aftercare.

In this chapter, we'll examine these points and many more. We know that when you ask your doctors the questions that we suggest, surgery may be avoided in many cases . . . and may never be needed. Most surgeries are elective. That means you have to decide if surgery is, in fact, the best option for you. Let's look at some of the key questions to ask prior to any surgery to keep you from making some potentially bad mistakes and reduce your risk of serious medical problems.

ARE THERE ANY OPTIONS OTHER THAN SURGERY?

Surgery is not without serious risks, no matter how common the procedure or how good the surgeon. Death is a very real possibility for high-risk surgeries like cardiac bypass surgery and abdominal aortic aneurysms, but is also a possibility even in simple surgeries like an appendectomy—albeit a remote one. Other problems that can occur with surgery are infections, lung problems, paralysis, and wound breakdowns, not to mention those associated with anesthesia.

As you've learned in the chapter about hospitals, just being in a hospital exposes a person to all sorts of potential risks like medication errors and hospital-acquired infections. As we've said, despite the best intentions of everyone involved in a surgical procedure, things can and do go wrong. The best doctors know that surgery should be a last option and utilized *only* after all other options have been exhausted. In some instances (and obviously in emergency situations), immediate surgery is both appropriate and necessary, but in the United States, most are elective. They don't have to be done right away but can be scheduled sometime in the future. This provides sufficient time for you to do your homework and to consider your alternatives.

Let's take as an example a very common surgery performed on many Baby Boomers as they age—hip replacement. This surgery is done all the time by many excellent surgeons. The success rates are exceptional, but the procedure is not without risk. Dick Schapp, the well-known sportscaster, died in 2001 of complications following what he thought was going to be routine hip replacement. He certainly knew of many other famous sports figures who had had similar surgeries with great success and few problems. He certainly didn't go into surgery thinking that anything would go wrong.

With every surgery you undergo, you are taking the chance that something can go wrong. Orthopedic surgeons who do frequent replacement procedures know this, and the good ones try to persuade their patients to wait as long as possible before undergoing surgery. Only when a patient has exhausted all other options, and can't take the pain any longer, do the best surgeons recommend surgery. Doctors know the same thing. We recommend strongly that you resort to surgery only as a last option.

Kevin's Comments

I had knee replacement surgery a couple of years ago at age fifty-five. Orthopedic doctors had advised me for years to put off surgery as long as possible because it wasn't without risk. They also told me that I would know when to get it done—when the quality of my life, or the pain, drove me to it. They were right, and fortunately, I had a good final result. But my surgery wasn't complication free. I lost so much blood in the leg that was operated on that I ended up needing a transfusion. This delayed my rehabilitation and physical therapy. I almost had to go back to surgery several weeks later because I couldn't bend my knee properly as a result of the initial problems. Luckily, my therapists really worked with me and no further surgery was needed, but it wasn't fun for quite a while. Remember, no surgery is without risk of complication . . . some more severe than others.

Explore your nonsurgical options with the doctor referring you to the surgeon as well as with the surgeon. Hopefully, between the primary care physician and the surgeon most alternatives to surgery will be known and can be explored. Don't depend on the referring physician alone to know something that may be outside the knowledge of his specialty. And some surgeons may not be familiar with options available for avoiding a particular surgery. It's incumbent upon you to do some of your own research by speaking to others with similar problems (like support groups), or by going on-line to research other choices.

Here's a very real scenario Kevin saw a lot of in the ER: A patient comes to the ER complaining of the sudden onset of severe pain in the right upper quadrant of the abdomen. After all the appropriate tests, he's diagnosed with an acute gallbladder attack (medically known as acute cholecystitis). A general surgeon is called and the patient is told that he probably should have his gallbladder removed as soon as it becomes less inflamed. He's admitted for a day or so and the pain disappears. Before having surgery, he does have some options. He could wait and see if he has another attack and then have surgery. He could also consider using oral medicines and making some dietary changes to reduce his risk of another attack. Finally, he could go ahead and have surgery. But even if he opts for surgery, there are choices to be made.

He can choose to have his gallbladder removed via conventional abdominal surgery or through a laparoscopic surgery. Laparoscopy is one of the biggest advances in what's known as minimally invasive surgery. During a laparoscopic procedure, the surgeon makes a tiny incision in the abdomen and uses a small scope to get to the gallbladder. Recovery time is only a few days and risks are minimal (the smaller incision means less blood loss, and the shorter time in the hospital reduces the chance of developing a hospital-acquired infection).

Conventional abdominal surgery, on the other hand, requires an incision going through your abdominal muscles to get to the inflamed gallbladder. Recovery time is considerably longer; you are disabled for four to six weeks. And there are many risks associated with opening your abdomen (serious infections and wounds not healing to mention a couple).

Why would anyone even consider conventional surgery? Well, maybe this is the only option the doctor recommends. Why? Not every surgeon is comfortable or skilled with the laparoscope. Laparoscopy is a relatively new procedure, and while younger surgeons learned this surgical technique in school, it wasn't available when older surgeons were training. They had to sign up for special courses to learn the technique or had to be trained by doctors already skilled in it. This is not to say that older surgeons cannot perform laparoscopy successfully, or are uncomfortable doing it. But this example should serve to encourage you to do some research and learn all your options.

Please understand that the majority of doctors have your best interest at heart and will inform you of all your options—surgical and nonsurgical. But remember, surgeons are trained to do surgery. Even when your primary care doctor refers you to a surgeon for her opinion, always ask about alternatives to surgery. Surgeons became surgeons because they are people of action and like to perform surgery. If something is wrong, most surgeons feel that surgery can help the situation. They are doers. There are many surgical axioms that support this point. One of the more famous: "When in doubt, cut it out."

Surgeons are often not taught much about the alternatives to surgery but figure you wouldn't have come to see them if you didn't want surgery. Wrong! As a patient, you want the doctor's opinion and advice about the options open to you to relieve your particular medical problem. Don't

Kevin's Comments

The single most important question to ask any doctor when he recommends a particular course of action (and especially in the case of surgery) is the following: "If your mother or your child had a similar problem, what would be the medical options you would give to them?" We have found this to be the most helpful question to ask other doctors. It never fails to provide important clues to the best possible treatment plan.

This is especially useful in cases involving heart problems. Often a patient who has a blockage of the coronary arteries has a variety of options. One could be coronary bypass surgery. Another might be angioplasty (placing a stent inside the arteries wall to hold it open), while a third might be medical management of the condition. There are pros and cons to each option (although in certain cases, there is only one correct choice). Nothing gets to the heart of the matter (pun intended) like asking the cardiologist and the cardiac surgeon what they would do if they or their family member had the problem. You may get a different answer from each, but you will get some real insights into the options.

assume that this is how your surgeon sees the situation. Always keep in mind that surgeons get paid when they operate. We don't want to give you the impression that they don't tell you the truth. They do. Many, however, believe that surgery is the answer to most problems. The best surgeons realize that this is definitely not always the case.

WHAT DOCTOR WOULD YOUR DOCTOR CHOOSE TO SEE?

Not all doctors are created equal. Some doctors are skilled in both the art of medicine (how they interact and relate to patients) and the science of medicine (the technical, scientific aspect), while others are much better at one or the other. The ideal doctor is one who possesses both the people skills and the technical skills. (We would gladly give up some people skills, if necessary, if we were facing a high-risk, technical procedure such as cardiac bypass surgery or neurosurgery. We want the surgeon who gets the best results.)

You should definitely ask your primary care doctor which doctor he or she would go to. When a doctor practices in a community or in a hospital for long enough, he or she quickly learns which doctors take the best care of their patients. Doctors come to know the strengths and weaknesses of their colleagues. They know whom they consider a good doctor and others that they wouldn't see unless there were few other choices. You should have this information too.

It is definitely fair to ask your doctor the following question: "If you were having the symptoms or problems that I am having, what doctor would you personally go see?" Make sure that the doctor with whom you are speaking understands that it does not necessarily have to be a doctor in the town in which you live, and the choice doesn't have to be limited by your insurance plan. Almost every doctor I know will give you an honest answer to this most important question. If the doctor you are asking becomes evasive or refuses to answer, then get another doctor. You can't trust him or her anyway.

Many people reading this book may not live in large metropolitan areas where there are multiple doctors to choose from in any given specialty. In this case, don't settle for convenience. The best surgeon or the best doctor to evaluate your problem may not be in the immediate area, but trust us, the drive is definitely worth it if your doctor tells you that he would go elsewhere. Do not take your doctor's recommendation lightly.

Finally, health insurance plans today often limit the number of doctors included in a given plan. They may not have all the specialists that a person might need. A plan may not include the best surgical groups because those surgeons refuse to settle for less money, especially when they do quality work and may actually be saving health insurance companies money in the long run. (Many insurance companies seem more concerned with saving money up front than with offering high-quality care that results in long-term savings.) The bottom line: You don't want to be limited by your insurance plan if the best surgeon for your particular situation is outside the plan. It might cost you more to go out of network, but money is not what it's all about when it comes to surgery.

If your insurance plan is limiting you, get the mortality and morbidity statistics and other health data on hospitals and surgeons that we mentioned in the chapter on hospitals. Use this to discover the differences between the surgeon you want and the surgeons in your plan. Then ask the insurance company how they can refuse you since you will have fewer complications and a lower risk of death.

HOW MANY OF THESE PARTICULAR SURGICAL PROCEDURES HAS THIS SURGEON PERFORMED?

The old axiom "practice makes perfect" may not always be true in surgery, but it definitely doesn't hurt. With any new skill—whether it be bike riding, skiing, video games, or tennis—it takes time to master the techniques required to be even average much less very good or comfortable. The same is true for surgery. It takes time for surgeons to learn new procedures and all the associated skills that go with them.

When surgeons study surgery in their residency, they learn many different procedures, but they are only learning those that are being done at that particular hospital and during that particular period of time. For instance, as little as ten years ago, few laparoscopic procedures were being done at certain hospitals. Today, a tremendous number of different laparoscopic procedures are being done. Surgeons who trained years ago have had to learn these new procedures or continue to do the old procedures. For instance, some gynecologists continue to perform total abdominal hysterectomies on their patients instead of doing the latest procedure, a laparoscopic-assisted vaginal hysterectomy. The reason? They feel uncomfortable doing a procedure for which they have not been trained. Unfortunately, it may be detrimental to their patients. In general, laparoscopic procedures allow patients to heal more quickly and avoid the trauma of abdominal surgery, with its associated risks of infection, adhesions, and increased pain.

For this reason, if your doctor suggests a particular surgical procedure for you, ask about alternative surgeries to accomplish this same end. Surgeries for weight loss in obese patients are a great example of a surgery that offers different options. There is a gastric bypass surgery using a laparoscope, and there's the same surgery that requires opening up the abdomen (old-style approach). There's a laparoscopic banding procedure of the stomach, and there's a mini-bypass procedure. What surgical procedure is right for each patient? The choice is often made by the doctor based on what she learned and what she feels comfortable doing. It's not that the other procedures aren't good, but the doctor has never learned them or she hasn't had experience with them. A particular surgery may not be best for you in your particular situation, so you need to ask your doctor why she has decided upon a particular method of surgery. Make sure to ask what your alternatives are. If your doctor doesn't do a particular type of surgery, you should consider consulting a doctor who does do it in order to learn the advantages of it. It might be money well spent for a second opinion.

Here's another example of why you need to know how many procedures

> If you have a choice (and you do in all elective surgeries), only allow surgeons who have lots of experience with your particular surgery to operate on you.

of a certain type your surgeon has done. One of our friends was referred to a reputable orthopedic group for a knee problem. He saw one of the doctors in the group who had a very good reputation. He was told that he had a problem requiring knee surgery. He had the surgery, but it had to be repeated six months later by another orthopedist. What he found out later was that the orthopedic doctor who first operated on him had only performed three knee operations in the past couple of years. He was a specialist in shoulders. He wasn't used to operating on knees, so he made some mistakes that don't occur when you perform a surgery regularly. If you have a choice (and you do in all elective surgeries), only allow surgeons who have lots of experience with your particular surgery to operate on you.

DO I REQUIRE A SURGICAL SPECIALIST FOR MY PARTICULAR TYPE OF SURGERY?

As we've said, not all surgeons are created equal. General surgeons are fine for most surgeries, but the data suggests that surgical specialists can definitely improve your chances of having a successful surgery, especially with complex, high-risk procedures. Death rates and complication rates are significantly lower for colorectal cancer operations when colorectal surgeons operate. This holds true when vascular surgeons perform abdominal aortic aneurysm surgery. Specialists are clearly better than general surgeons when it comes to high-risk surgical procedures. They have more training and they perform these procedures more frequently. Practice generally makes for a better outcome.

The field of medicine is constantly changing, and surgery is no exception. The way we do cardiac bypass procedures has changed tremendously over the years. Nowadays it's faster, safer, and takes advantage of new technology. Surgeons have to keep up with these constant changes or be left behind. If they don't keep up, they may put their patients at increased risk of surgical complications. Surgeons learn these new techniques and how to utilize the latest technology by going to continuing medical education (CME) courses, by training with other doctors, and by reading. To maintain licensure, states and most medical specialties require a specific number of CME hours every year or every couple of years. It's a good idea to check to see if your doctor maintains his or her ongoing education. If not, get out of that office fast. (Ask the state medical licensing board to confirm that the doctor has done the required CME coursework. You can also ask the office staff if the doctor ever takes time off to go to CME courses.)

WHAT IS THE BEST HOSPITAL FOR MY PARTICULAR SURGICAL PROCEDURE?

In Chapter 4, we clearly outlined the importance of picking the right hospital to have a particular surgical procedure. The data is very clear on this. Please do your research.

The data clearly demonstrates that a hospital must perform a certain minimum number of cardiac bypass surgical procedures to be able to reduce the complication rate associated with that particular type of surgery. (See Chapter 4 for more information on the volume of surgeries and the risk of problems.) If a hospital doesn't perform this minimum number, your chances of dying in surgery can almost double. It takes time for the hospital staff and surgical teams to become proficient at supporting high-risk surgical procedures of any type. Like any of us, if we don't do something frequently enough, we tend to make mistakes when we do it, or we don't do whatever it is as well.

How do you find out if your hospital is up to par? We think there are two ways to discover this information. First, find out the complication rate from your hospital for your particular surgical procedure, and second, go to the HealthGrades Web site to research this information. (See Chapter 4 again.)

WHAT HOSPITAL HAS THE BEST ANESTHESIOLOGISTS?

Besides your surgeon, who do you think is the most important person on your surgical team? We believe that your anesthesiologist may be the most critical supporting player on your team. Anesthesiologists are doctors who are responsible for putting you to sleep safely in surgery (and waking you up of course), and monitoring your vital signs, your breathing, and the way your heart functions during surgery. Depending on the individual case, anesthesiologists also provide regional anesthesia (anesthetizing only the part of the body that will undergo surgery) or sedation for surgical procedures that are performed under local anesthesia.

Fortunately, anesthesia, general or regional, is safer than it's ever been. In 1980, the death rates due to anesthesia were 1 in 10,000. Today it's improved dramatically to 1 in 250,000 people. Much of the improvement has occurred as increasingly better monitors of heart, lung, and brain function have become available for use in the operating room. There are still risks associated with anesthesia. If too little anesthesia is used, there can be problems during surgery (patients have actually awakened and felt pain). If too much is used, there can be problems recovering after surgery (you can sleep too long and can then develop breathing problems or increase your risk of pneumonia). It was common practice in the past to have other physicians not specifically trained in anesthesia put patients to sleep, but now, fortunately for us all, this is rare. It's another big reason why the safety record in anesthesia has improved over the years.

Your anesthesia team (we say "anesthesia team" because getting put to sleep is often a team effort in many hospitals) will most likely consist of an anesthesiologist (a doctor who has done a residency in anesthesia) and a nurse anesthetist (a nurse who takes additional training to be certified in anesthesia). What you want from an anesthesia team is that they consider all aspects of your health and use the optimal combination of drugs to get you through surgery safely and as pain free as possible. Your team should prepare you in advance so that your chances of suffering any adverse events are minimized.

The anesthesiologist (the doctor) should be present at all the critical points in the surgical process, if not more often. Although nurse anesthetists practice in some hospitals without supervision by a physician anesthesiologist, it is important to remember that physician anesthesiologists undergo four years of medical school training after college and at least four years of anesthesiology residency after medical school. In contrast, nurse anesthetists train only for about three years after nursing school.

The nurse anesthetist often monitors the patient during the routine parts of surgery. The most critical times in any surgery are when you're first being put to sleep in case there's an emergency, and when you emerge from sleep and have the breathing tube used during surgery removed. Your anesthesiologist makes sure that only those persons with medical training make medical decisions. We wouldn't want it any other way.

How do you determine who is the best anesthesiologist or anesthesia team? In general, it is best to choose a board-certified anesthesiologist. Board certification means that an anesthesiologist has passed both a rigorous written examination and an intense oral examination by experts. It is also reassuring to know that an anesthesiologist has voluntarily taken the written test to become recertified if their original certification is more than ten years old.

When we asked anesthesiologists about finding the best anesthesia team, their answers were always the same: "Ask your surgeon. He or she will always know who the best people are as well as those to avoid." Another way to find out if there are anesthesiologists to avoid is to ask your hospital if there are any lawsuits against any anesthesia team members. Hospitals cannot afford to put themselves at risk with a poor anesthesiologist or anesthetist because it can cost them millions in lawsuits. Finally, the Joint Commission on Accreditation of Hospitals requires that all hospitals seeking accreditation keep quality-assurance statistics on the outcomes and complications (including anesthesia) associated with surgical procedures.

Because the anesthesiologist is so crucial to the ultimate success of your surgery, it is important that you have the opportunity to meet with him or her before surgery. How can your anesthetist assess you adequately, and how care you assess her understanding of your unique body and mental makeup, if you never meet? What doctors know is that you need to meet with a member of your anesthesia team to help determine the best anesthesia for you. No meeting with the anesthesiologist (either by phone or in person), no surgery. Period! Of course we're only talking about elective surgery here because you may not be in any condition to speak to someone in emergency surgery . . . and that's one of the reasons people are at increased risk in emergency situations.

Christine's Comments

I was scheduled for a simple surgical procedure. The surgeon assured me that it was a routine outpatient procedure that would only require local anesthesia and that I'd be going home only hours after the procedure was complete.

I was scheduled for the procedure at the last minute due to an opening in my surgeon's busy schedule and I was told that for minor outpatient surgical procedures, anesthesiologists did not do consults. A red flag went up in my head. I thought, "I don't care what the policy is, I really want to talk to him." But because I was nervous about the upcoming surgery, I didn't press the point and ignored my intuition (see even doctors make mistakes!)

The morning of the surgery, the anesthesiologist showed up in a patient bay where I was one of several patients waiting for surgery. He walked in, barely looked at me, and said that he was going to start my general anesthesia.

When I protested and told him that my surgeon and I had discussed in great detail that all I would be needing was local anesthesia, he told me I was mistaken, and we had to get on without because he was in a hurry and had other patients to get to. Well, you can bet that didn't set well with me. No way was I going to let this anesthesiologist, who clearly did not know my case, and who had not adequately reviewed my chart, do anything to me. I decided right there to refuse anesthesia and cancel my surgery.

Bottom line: It is as important to meet, interview and trust your anesthesiologist as it is to know and trust your surgeon. Unless you are in an ER and have no choice, make sure that you take the very important step of interviewing your anesthesiologist before having any surgical procedure—major or minor.

The most important thing that your anesthesia team must do prior to surgery is to take a good medical history from you. How else will they know the medicines you are taking, your allergies, your previous reactions to anesthesia, your fears or concerns, or your special needs? If this doesn't happen in person or through a good phone interview, don't have your surgery until it does. It's just too important. No doctor would get put to sleep unless he talked with a member of the anesthesia team prior to surgery, and neither should you.

An informed, relaxed patient is an easier patient and requires less medicine during and after surgery. Besides providing honest answers to the questions on your medical history (some people don't and it hurts them at times), the other way that you can help reduce your risk from surgery and from getting anesthesia is to express any fears or concerns you might have. Are you scared of being put to sleep because you're afraid that you might not wake up again? If you've heard horror stories about spinal anesthesia causing someone to become paralyzed or have severe headaches for years, air your concerns. The anesthesiologist isn't a mind reader. Tell her straight out, "I have a fear of . . ." Your anesthesia team is there to help, but they need information only you can provide.

Follow the instructions you are given by the anesthetist prior to surgery to the letter, especially when it involves children. Failure to follow presurgical instructions has put many patients at considerable risk. Let's share a few examples. A mother is told to give her child nothing to eat or drink after midnight in preparation for surgery early in the morning. The child is crying and complaining the next morning, so the mother gives him some juice or milk. What happens next? The child gets sick and nauseous thanks to the anesthesia, throws up, and then gets the juice or milk in his lungs (the medical term for this is aspiration), causing all kinds of serious problems. NBO (nothing by mouth) means just that . . . NOTHING BY MOUTH. This is the rule that seems to be broken most often. If the doctor says take any pills with a sip of water, take as little water as possible to get the pills down. If the doctor tells you to stop medicines three days prior to surgery, then do this. Failing to follow the doctor's instructions just puts you at risk for complications that can mean your life or permanent medical injury. Why take the chance? Doctors know that these instructions are there for a reason . . . you should too.

There's one more important point to consider when it comes to your anesthesia. There is a significant shortage of both anesthesiologists and nurse anesthetists today. It's gotten so bad that some hospitals can't fully staff operating rooms. A Cleveland Clinic study indicates that about four thousand more anesthesiologists are needed to meet the demand. This shortage puts tremendous pressure on existing anesthesia personnel. Experiments using simulated (robot) patients clearly show that sleep-deprived anesthesiologists can make some dangerous mistakes. The drugs that are given during surgery are not without risk and can kill people if not monitored properly. So what should you do? Ask about the staffing at your hospital and find out what kind of shifts these specialists are pulling before deciding on the best place for your surgery.

IF SURGERY CAN'T BE AVOIDED, WHAT CAN I PERSONALLY DO TO HELP REDUCE MY RISK OF PROBLEMS DURING AND AFTER SURGERY?

We've been emphasizing the importance of choosing the best hospital, surgeon, and support staff for your surgery. And in fact, doing the research and making informed choices can literally be a matter of life and death. But a patient's attitude and general health play a major role in the success of surgery.

Be Honest With Your Doctor

Above all, the most important thing you can do prior to surgery is to honestly communicate to your doctor your medical history, medicines, personal habits, and lifestyle. Here's a scenario we've seen all too frequently in practice. A doctor asks a question about a person's habits or medicines and a patient fails to give an honest or accurate answer. It's hard to believe that patients would mislead or lie to their doctors when their very life might be on the line, but it happens all too often. We've seen it ourselves in our practices. Doctors ask the questions they do for very specific reasons. If you are a smoker, your lungs may be at greater risk after anesthesia than those of a nonsmoker, so your respiratory system may require more attention. It's amazing how often patients lie about their smoking habits when doctors ask.

Some patients fail to tell doctors when they have breathing problems like asthma or if they have other medical problems that are intermittent in nature but can affect their overall health. It makes no sense to hide medical information from your doctor, because if things go wrong, or if your condition should flare up again, it will take longer for your doctor to make the correct diagnosis. By concealing information for whatever reason, you could be given the wrong medicine or wrong treatment, and these can make your condition worse. Don't hide information or omit things from your medical history no matter how personal or embarrassing. Your doctor needs this to help you.

It is your responsibility to inform your surgeon of the medicines you are taking, and it's his responsibility to ask about all the medicines you are taking. It's important to mention all medicines, vitamins, or supplements that you are taking to all your doctors because they will likely want to continue these medicines while you are in the hospital. In the case of cardiac medicines, it is extremely important that these drugs not be discontinued without consulting a physician or serious medical problems can occur. There are numerous cases in which surgeons are not aware of certain medicines that patients are taking prior to surgery, and because of this, the surgeon fails to write the necessary orders postoperatively to continue the medicines. Just imagine if you were a diabetic or had high blood pressure and you didn't take your medicines. Nothing good can come of it.

Some medicines should be stopped prior to surgery—but not abruptly. They must be slowly tapered off to lessen the problems for the patient. If your doctor is not aware of the medicines you are taking, he won't be able to counsel you appropriately on how to stop your medicines. *(When I had knee replacement surgery, they advised me to stop my anti-inflammatory drug at least one week prior to surgery to lessen the chances of bleeding problems during the surgery—Kevin.)*

YOUR MEDICATIONS AND SURGERY MAY MAKE FOR A FATAL MIX

Don't assume that your primary care doctor and your surgeon ever communicate about the medications you are taking prior to your surgery. Continuing certain medicines or combinations of medicines prior to surgery can negatively interact with anesthesia medications and even increase your chances of dying in surgery. Taking anti-inflammatory medications may increase your chances of bleeding during and after surgery. For instance, if you are taking a baby aspirin every day to reduce your risk of heart attack or stroke, this may need to be stopped a few days prior to surgery as aspirin can increase bleeding during and after an operation if your doctor also gives you a blood thinner to prevent problems after surgery. You also need to inform your doctors about any over-the-counter vitamin or herbal supplements you might be taking. Make it your responsibility to see your primary care physician prior to surgery and get his or her recommendations about medications. You can then take these suggestions to your surgeon, or you should insist that your PCP talk or write a note to your surgeon discussing your medications.

You also should ask your PCP to check on you while you're in the hospital. He or she should be the primary manager of all the care that is *not* related to surgery. Someone needs to coordinate the care that you get in the hospital. Trust us, most surgeons are not good at this. They care about surgery. There's an old joke about this. "The surgery went well but the patient died." Your PCP should oversee your care. He or she should make sure the entire team communicates about your health and everyone knows what everyone else is doing so that the whole team works together to give you the best possible care.

Make Lifestyle Changes to Increase Surgery Success

Most people, when they actually think about how they might be able to reduce risk during surgery, think about specific health-related actions. This makes sense especially when we think about the health risks that get most people in trouble before surgery: alcohol and tobacco use.

Anything that you can do to stop or cut down your smoking prior to surgery can have a positive effect on your health. Smokers develop problems both during and after surgery more than nonsmokers because their lungs are not as elastic and they often have underlying pulmonary or lung disease. During and following surgery, when patients are in one position in bed, their normal secretions pool in the most "dependent" part of their lungs and are a perfect setup for pneumonia. Stopping smoking as soon as you can prior to surgery will begin to help your lungs to heal and begin clearing some of the toxins from them. Despite these facts, many people can't or don't stop smoking prior to surgery. Smoking is a major health risk in surgery, so we advise you to do whatever you can to stop.

A big problem contributing to disability and even death after surgery is alcohol use that your surgeon or anesthesiologist is unaware of. Alcohol use can produce problems after surgery because patients who drink regularly and are dependent on alcohol often develop a condition known as delirium tremens or the DTs. It can take as little as a couple of drinks per week to put some people into this potentially dangerous situation. It can increase your risk of seizures, hallucinations, and breathing problems.

What can you do? Stop all alcohol well before surgery and be sure to tell your doctor the truth about your use of alcohol.

Increasing your physical activity is also a good thing to do prior to surgery if you are physically able to do so. It will increase your muscle tone, improve your breathing, and stimulate your cardiovascular system. All these are positive factors for your health and will lessen your risk of problems following surgery.

The Mind, the Emotions, and Surgical Success

There is significant support in the medical literature for the use of psychological interventions to improve surgical outcomes. Unfortunately, surgical programs rarely focus on the mind-body connection but instead emphasize the technical aspects of surgery to the exclusion of almost everything else. The best surgeons (and the best teachers) understand that there is an art to surgery. They also understand and promote the role of psychoneuroimmunology (the mind-body-spirit) connection in the ultimate successful outcomes of their patients.

Dr. Curt Tribble is the head of thoracic surgery at the University of Virginia and performs coronary bypass procedures (CABG) on very sick patients. Because their underlying heart disease is so severe, they have no other choice but to have this very serious surgical procedure, which includes a very real risk of death. Patients facing this surgery are scared, and it causes every one of them to reflect on their lives prior to their operation. Dr. Tribble knows this and asks every person to help him through surgery in a very unique way.

Prior to surgery, Dr. Tribble asks, "What do you personally want to be able to do after your successful surgery? What activity is the most important in your life that you will miss the most and want to return to?" What he's found is that most people want to return to the simple things like playing with their grandchildren, going fishing, puttering in the garden, or watching sunsets. Most of his patients want nothing fancy—just the chance to experience the special times in their lives. When he discovers what his patients most want to do following surgery—their dream—he asks them to concentrate and think about their dream prior to surgery, during surgery, and following surgery. He asks them to leave all the worrying about surgery to him, since he is the specialist, and instead, concentrate on their dream. What he finds is that this relaxes his patients and that they are better able to concentrate and work on their recovery. It enables his patients to participate in their surgery and, he feels, reduces problems after surgery.

Let us review a few of the psychoneuroimmunology studies because we believe it's so important yet so poorly utilized. Suggestion, relaxation, and hypnosis in surgery have resulted in shorter hospital stays and fewer postoperative complications. Plastic surgery patients who underwent hypnosis showed significant reductions in pain, postoperative nausea and vomiting, postoperative anxiety, and overall satisfaction. Women undergoing elective breast reduction surgery who underwent preoperative hypnosis and mental preparation had less nausea, less vomiting, and a reduced need for pain control. Patients undergoing elective colorectal surgical procedures were able to reduce postoperative pain medications by almost 50 percent by using positive imaging techniques. Need we say more?

It's all about the end results, so if your surgeon doesn't use or recommend some of these techniques, it might be useful to see a psychologist to help teach you some of the mental techniques and to put you in the right frame of mind for your surgery.

WHAT ABOUT USING REHABILITATION OR PHYSICAL THERAPY AFTER SURGERY?

One of the biggest failings of many surgeons is not guiding their patients into an aggressive rehabilitation or physical therapy plan following surgery. Wouldn't you agree that the primary goal of most patients is getting back to their previous state of health or functioning following surgery? The best way to do this is to follow your surgeon's orders, but a part of your return to health should be a rehabilitation plan specific for you. Obviously, not all surgeries require a rehabilitation plan, but many patients would profit from a postop plan that included big doses of therapy designed to restore the functioning of their body, mind, and spirit.

Kevin's Comments

I have played many sports throughout my life at a highly competitive level. As a consequence, I have suffered many injuries that have required many surgeries (eight major surgeries to be specific . . . but who's counting?). My two most recent surgeries have been a knee replacement and a rotator cuff repair of my shoulder. I can now do anything that I want to do physically (within reason for my age) and I'm in much less pain than I was prior to surgery. My surgeons did an excellent job, but what really got me back functioning again was the intensive, long physical therapy that I went through for each of these surgeries. My therapists helped me to do the really hard work that it took to make my surgery a success.

While I was at the physical therapist's doing my exercises and my therapy for my knee, I saw many other patients who had also had knee replacements. Most had been sent by their doctors while a handful of others came on their own. What surprised me the most was that many doctors never referred their patients to therapy after having joint replacement surgery. This was shocking to me. Knowing what I was going through, I wondered how anyone could ever get back to almost normal functioning again without therapy. The patients who weren't sent to therapy probably wouldn't get the full benefit from the major surgery they had just gone through.

I bet if any of these same doctors ever had joint replacement surgery themselves, they would be the first ones in line for physical therapy. Not recommending therapy often joint surgery seems almost like malpractice to me and still amazes me today. Why wouldn't you at least offer it to patients? How can you not do for your patients what you would want done for yourself?

Cardiovascular Rehabilitation Following Heart Surgery

The great cardiologist Dr. Paul Dudley White was one of the early leaders in his field. When he spoke to other doctors, he advocated treatment of the total patient—their mind, their body, and their spirit. He would explain that doctors couldn't just take care of a patient's heart, but had to understand their total needs. If a doctor failed to take care of a patient's emotional state following a heart attack, the patient might do poorly even if their heart was in good shape. Over the forty years since Dr. White first began espousing this view, more and more physicians have come to this same understanding.

Rehabilitation of the cardiovascular system is one of the more frequently underutilized therapies, but you'd better believe that the majority of physicians would ask for it if they had heart complications. The data from many studies clearly shows that people undergoing cardiac rehabilitation live longer and have a better quality of life than those who fail to go through a rehab program.

Cardiac rehab is beneficial for patients with a variety of cardiac problems and should not be limited to those who have had heart attacks or bypass surgery. Those benefiting from cardiac rehab include people having the following:

- Congestive heart failure

- Angina

- Coronary artery bypass surgery (CABG)

- Myocardial infarction (MI) or heart attack

- PCTA (balloon angioplasty)

- Pacemakers

- Congenital cardiovascular disease

Because of this, the American Heart Association has outlined some principles of cardiac rehabilitation that focus on the total patient. They are as follows:

- Patients should be counseled about their understanding of the disease process and its management.

- An exercise program should be an integral part of any cardiac rehab program.

- Modifiable risk factors for cardiac disease and stroke should be altered and modified. Patients should gain an understanding of how these risk factors impact their chances of living or having a quality life.

- Vocational guidance should be provided to enable patients to work if they so desire.

- Physical limitations should be addressed as best as possible.

■ Emotional support and counseling should be an important program component.

■ Patients should be assessed initially and regularly after the precipitating event for depression, anxiety, distress, dependence, or inadequate social support.

■ Patient compliance should be closely monitored, as long-term success is totally dependent on patient involvement.

By paying attention to these basic principles, a cardiac rehab program can improve the functional capacity of patients, can enhance the quality of life, and create a sense of well-being and optimism about the future. Our advice to you: Make sure that your doctor refers you or your family member to a good cardiovascular rehabilitation program. After that, it's up to you to take advantage of this life-improving therapy.

Second Opinions and Surgery

Many health plans insist on second opinions when surgery is being considered in order to help prevent unneeded surgeries. In most cases, the second opinions confirm the need for surgery, but what should you do if what the second surgeon suggests is different from the first? Here are some things you can or consider:

Get a third opinion. It can be hard to find three doctors who practice separately in smaller towns, so you may have to travel to get another opinion, but it can be worth the trouble. Your insurer can often help you find a doctor who has good credentials. Another option is to check with friends and see what doctors they've been pleased with in the past. If two of the three agree, then that's generally the best decision.

Trust your intuition. Most people never go wrong when they trust their own instincts. The difficult part is taking the time and focusing on your inner voice. All doctors won't agree, so if you have to make a choice, trust yourself.

Go with the teachers. If you are getting an opinion from a surgeon who works in a teaching hospital and another from one who does not, you may want to give more weight to the opinion of the former. Why? The staff in teaching hospitals is more likely to keep up with the latest research, the latest procedures, and the pros and cons of various surgeries.

More is better. As we said earlier, the surgeon who does the procedure more frequently and works with the same team is more likely to have better results. She is also more likely to understand the pros and cons of that surgery and be able to determine who would benefit most from the operation as well.

Think conservatively. If one surgeon recommends a more conservative approach, then that might be a better option to consider. Being too aggressive may not be needed. Be careful of doctors who have a large staff to support or extremely opulent-looking offices. Someone has to pay for this overhead, so you may get more surgery than is really needed. This is not always true, but it should send up warning flags for you.

WHAT DOCTORS KNOW ABOUT
Surgery . . . And You Should Too

Doctors know that having surgery is not without risk and that both the hospital and the surgeon you choose are integral to the ultimate success of the operation. Asking your surgeon some key questions before surgery will improve your chances for a successful surgery. And don't forget, rehabilitation is an important part of your ultimate recovery back to normal function.

Ten Questions to Ask Your Surgeon Before Surgery

1. What are the risks of delaying surgery or trying a nonsurgical approach to treatment prior to surgery? This is, are there any other options to surgery?

2. If your doctor were having this surgery, whom would they get to do it?

3. How many of the same procedures has the surgeon I am considering done?

4. Which hospital has the team best skilled in this type of procedure and how many of these surgeries have they done?

5. What are the most common complications associated with this surgery at this hospital and with this surgeon?

6. What are my choices for anesthesia for this surgery? What are the pros and cons of each?

7. What can I do prior to surgery to make myself more ready and increase my chances for success?

8. What medicines should I stop prior to surgery and when should I stop them?

9. What type of rehabilitation therapy should I have after surgery?

10. Should I get a second opinion?

CHAPTER SIX

DRUGS,
PHARMACOGENOMICS,
AND VITAMINS

Do you ever wonder why some people take a drug and seem to get no bene-fit while others take the same dose and develop serious side effects? Do women have different side effects than men? Are you aware of a little-known killer in medicine that takes the lives of 100,000 people every year, yet is rarely talked about? Why are some antibiotics not as effective as they used to be? Why are physicians concerned about the development of "super bugs" that might be resistant to all available antibiotics? Do you know why not telling your health care provider about all the medicines, over-the-counter drugs, vitamins, and supplements you might be taking could put your life at risk?

These are a few of the questions and issues that will be addressed in this chapter. Some of what you learn may disturb and shock you . . . and it should. You are potentially putting yourself and your loved ones at risk by not knowing this critical information.

1. Adverse drug events are a major threat to patients that is often unrecognized and unappreciated by doctors and patients.

2. Women can be more at risk from serious medication side effects than men.

3. Different people require different doses of a drug based on age and their individual ability to metabolize drugs.

4. Direct advertising to consumers can generate sales of expensive medicines that are not needed.

5. Many bacteria today are developing resistance to common antibiotics because doctors and patients are overusing antibiotics.

6. Many people overuse vitamins while others don't take enough.

7. Supplements have side effects and can interfere with medicines that people are taking.

ADVERSE DRUG EVENTS: THE LITTLE-KNOWN KILLER

Do you know the name of the killer that takes the life of more than twice the number of women who die from breast cancer each year? It's a little-known killer that medical professionals call adverse drug events. Adverse drug events (ADEs) are problems that cause over 2 million hospital admissions a year and over 100,000 deaths in the United States alone. You are more likely to die from a medication error than you are from an automobile accident, a gunshot wound, or a stroke. The market for the necessary services and products needed to solve this massive problem is estimated to

> Adverse drug events (ADEs) are problems that cause over 2 million hospital admissions a year and over 100,000 deaths in the U.S. alone

be $14 billion by 2010. The National Association of Chain Drug Stores reported that we spend $142 billion annually on prescription drugs—then spend $177 billion to fix the medication errors that send us to the hospital.

Here's a statistic that shocked us and will get your attention as well. A recent study of thirty-six U.S. hospitals and skilled nursing facilities found that one in five times at a typical three-hundred-bed hospital—19 percent of the time—medication doses given were in error. Seven percent of these errors had the potential for causing an adverse drug event as judged by an outside panel of experts. In a nutshell, these errors represent more than forty potential adverse drug effects per day in a three-hundred-patient facility. Errors included wrong doses, doses being omitted or given at the wrong time, and an unauthorized drug being given.

How can these mistakes happen? It can be as simple as a doctor's writing being illegible. Imagine the havoc that bad penmanship could cause with the following three look-alike and sound-alike prescription drugs:

Celebrex: an oral, nonsteroidal anti-inflammatory medication used to treat pain from arthritis

Celexa: an oral, selective serotonin reuptake inhibitor used to treat depression

Cerebyx: a parenteral anticonvulsant drug

If you say the names of these medications out loud, they sound alike. If you write the prescription and your handwriting is less than perfect, it would be easy for a pharmacy to make an error. It is easy to see how taking the wrong medication might lead to serious complications. One of the best solutions to prevent this problem: Doctors enter the prescription medications that they want to order for a patient into a computer system instead of depending on writing anything down longhand. It's a simple solution that can prevent deadly medication errors, but for reasons of cost, not all doctors offices or hospitals are willing to invest in the necessary computer systems.

What can you do to protect you and your family? Know the medicines that you are being given and question the nurse each time you are given something to make sure it's correct. If you have a family member whose mind may be affected by health or medications, post the medicines and dosages on their bed above their head as a constant reminder to medical professionals.

What more can hospitals do to reduce the risk of deadly adverse drug effects? In March 2003, the Food and Drug Administration (FDA) decided to step in. By the spring of 2004, their proposal will ensure that every medication given in a hospital carries a label with the same supermarket-style bar codes that you see on cereal, milk, and magazines. These bar codes will ensure that patients get the right dose of the right drug at the right time. An estimated seven thousand hospitalized patients die annually because of drug errors, where either the wrong dose or the wrong drug is dispensed. When the FDA's proposed bar-code rule is enacted, it could prevent more than 400,000 health problems in the first twenty years it is in place.

Here's how bar codes could help save lives: When you are admitted to a hospital that uses bar-code scanners, you will receive an ID bracelet with a bar code linked to your medical records. Every drug label will have a bar code signifying its unique National Drug Code number, which serves to identify the medication, its dosage form, and strength. Before giving you any drug, a nurse will scan its bar code as well as the bar code on your ID bracelet. The bar code will verify if you are getting the right drug in the right dose and in the right formulation. According to the FDA, the hospitals that are already using bar-code technology have seen their medication error rates drop by more than 70 percent.

Until these new, national guidelines are implemented, some definite precautions can still be taken to reduce adverse drug effects in the hospital setting and you should check to see if your hospital has them in place. If it does not, you need to be even more cautious about the medications you are receiving while in the hospital. Does your hospital have:

- Computerized prescription error notification systems?

- Pharmacists who screen medication orders for allergies, drug interactions, and inappropriate medicine doses?

- Clinical practice guidelines that aid in prescribing?

- Pharmacists who consult with physicians about their patients who have kidney or liver problems that could alter the dose of medicines used?

- Scannable bar coding on all medication packages and containers?

Medication errors and adverse drug effects should be considered system failures, so having the right system in place can help eliminate most errors of this type. One study in the *American Journal of Health System-Pharmacy* found that including a pharmacist on daily patient rounds cut medication errors by about 50 percent. Why not ask your hospital to make these changes? No matter what the excuse, if they're not in place, lobby for the changes. After all, it could be your life, or the life of a loved one.

WHAT ARE ADVERSE DRUG EVENTS?

An adverse drug event (ADE) can be simply defined as a person having a reaction to a drug that his or her body can't tolerate. The pharmaceutical industry is well aware of these adverse drug effects because they have to document them in the fine print of their ads in magazines (if you can read them, you don't need to see your doctor for an eye exam because you've got remarkable vision) or mention them oh-so-quickly at the end of television commercials. These adverse drug effects are not a new problem and most of us know someone who has had a negative reaction, however minor, to some drug that they've been taking. Here are a few examples of adverse drug effects:

- Your child becomes hyperactive or you lie awake all night after taking an OTC cold medication.

- You develop crampy abdominal pain after taking the antibiotic erythromycin.

- A cough develops after taking a particular class of high blood pressure medicines.

- Your liver is affected after taking high doses of acetaminophen.

- You develop bleeding from your rectum after taking nonsteroidal anti-inflammatory (NSAID) medicines for your arthritis.

These are not unusual problems, as they affect thousands of people on a daily basis. When you take a medicine or drug, you can have three possible reactions:

1. It works as intended and your health improves.

2. Nothing happens and the physician changes to a new drug, ups the dose of your present drug, or adds another drug.

3. There is a mild, moderate, or serious adverse drug reaction.

Kevin's Comments

I take a prescription NSAID drug for arthritis in my back and knees every day and have been doing this for years. I tried other medicines in this group of drugs, but I had some stomach upset with them, so my personal physician switched me to a newer version of an NSAID that is less upsetting to my stomach. It works very well and I don't have any problems with it at this time.

Being over fifty, I decided one day to begin taking a baby aspirin every day to help reduce my risk of heart attack and stroke. I advise my patients to do this, so why shouldn't I do the same thing? About four or five days after beginning the baby aspirin, I noticed some blood on my handkerchief when I blew my nose. I didn't think anything about it because it was winter and I figured that my nose was dried out because of indoor heat and the little amount of moisture in the air. Two days later, while I was at work, blood started to pour out of my nose. I tried everything I knew to stop the bleeding, but it was no good. I was swallowing blood down the back of my throat.

I called one of my ENT (ear, nose, and throat) doctor friends, who saw me immediately in his office. He quickly found a bleeding blood vessel in my nose, put some medicine on it to stop the bleeding, and then packed my nose for forty-eight hours. When we talked about what the problem might be, he inquired about all the medicines I was taking. I told him that all I was taking was my NSAID and the baby aspirin. "Bingo," he said. "The combination of drugs is what caused your nose to bleed." The light bulb went on then. I knew he was correct.

Since then, I've never taken aspirin again in combination with my other drug and I've never had another nosebleed. You see, it can even happen to doctors. Sometimes, we don't think about what we do and it causes a drug reaction. I learned a good lesson that day and will definitely keep my patients from making the same mistake I made.

Some drug reactions are relatively harmless, just inconvenient and uncomfortable—like trouble sleeping. But this isn't always the case. The problem that all doctors have is that they can't predict how a patient may or may not react to any medicine that they prescribe . . . at least not yet.

ARE WOMEN MORE AT RISK THAN MEN FROM MEDICINES?

Women may be more at risk from potentially life-threatening side effects from medications than are men. In the case of eight of the ten medicines that the FDA pulled off the market since 1997, women suffered more serious side effects. Researchers found that more problems with medicines occurred in women even though ten times as many men were taking the drugs.

There is a gender-specific reason why women may react differently. Women seem to metabolize drugs differently than men do, and it may be because male hormones make men less sensitive to drugs. Another reason for the difference in drug reactions is the muscle-to-fat ratio of women versus men. Women have more fat, and because drugs are often stored in fat, they react differently within a woman's body.

How come this "gender bias" in side effects wasn't noticed before? There are many reasons. Until 1972, women of childbearing age weren't even allowed to participate in clinical trials of medications. Even now, side effects that are noted in studies are often not differentiated by sex. And because reporting of side effects is voluntary for doctors, it's estimated that the FDA learns about only 10 percent of side effects. Without this information, it's hard to provide proper drug warnings for both men and women.

Of the ten drugs pulled off the market since 1997, only two had warnings about specific effects in women. Doctors just don't know how many medicines will react in men versus women. Right now, it's often a guessing game. Ask your doctor what side effects are most common to specific medication before you start on it. Pay close attention to any changes in your body when you begin taking it and report these to your doctor.

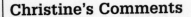

Christine's Comments

Several years ago, my heart started to race for no apparent reason, as if I had been running sprints. My doctor ultimately found out that it was simple acid reflux that was causing this reaction. In the meantime, though, I had every possible heart test taken and each one said that my heart was 100 percent healthy. I had cardiologists and ER physicians perplexed from coast to coast.

Before the mystery was solved, one cardiologist thought that a beta-blocker medication might help my problem. He wrote a prescription dose that I knew was more appropriate for a large male with a cardiac problem, which, of course, they had no evidence that I had. I suggested to the cardiologist that the dosage was too high for my five-foot three-inch female frame. His response to me: "Who is the cardiologist?" My intuition told me that I was correct. I am the daughter of a pharmacist and I learned about drug names and dosages the way other kids learned the alphabet. But this important cardiologist intimidated even me. So I had the prescription filled and I took the dose that he prescribed.

About forty-eight hours later, I started feeling very ill. Fortunately, I was at my parents' home at the time, and not alone when it happened. I told them to call 911. They called the paramedics, and as I waited for them to come, I thought to myself, "This must be what it feels like right before you die." By the time the paramedics came, my blood pressure had dropped to about 60/35. They took me to a hospital ER, and I was fortunate enough to survive the medication error incident and to have a happy ending.

Lesson learned: Women are not like men. We need different dosages of drugs and sometimes physicians don't realize this.

Also, I learned, the hard way, to trust my intuition. The cardiologist was giving me too much medicine. I knew it and he intimidated me into overriding my instincts. It almost cost me my life. It will never happen again.

FLYING BY THE SEAT OF YOUR PANTS

Currently, in almost all cases, physicians and pharmaceutical companies rely on guesswork when it comes to detecting how a specific patient will react to a particular medicine. There are no tests that will help us predict who will respond to a drug and who won't. Basically, it's trial-and-error medicine. We doctors are playing the odds. When we give you a drug, we are betting that you will fall into the vast majority of patients who react normally and get the intended benefit without serious side effects. We are betting that you won't have a severe reaction.

Because there are so many medications on the market today (over seventeen thousand) and there are a multitude of side effects associated with each one, physicians cannot possibly know every instance in which a patient may have an ADE. In many cases, in the hope of discovering problems with a drug or drugs, a physician will ask a patient a general question about how they're doing. This often does not generate much in the way of beneficial information. Instead, physicians should be asking very pointed questions about specific side effects patients might be experiencing. This problem only gets compounded when a patient is taking multiple medications. How can your doctor possibly know when you are having a drug reaction unless you tell him or her how you're feeling, and how you have changed since beginning a particular medicine? Only you know how you're feeling, so tune in to yourself. Then make a list of your concerns or how you're feeling differently, and speak to your doctor about them at each visit.

There are some classic drug reactions and most physicians know about

10 Critical Questions to Ask Before Taking Any Prescription Medication

Here are the questions that every patient needs to ask their doctor and their pharmacist when they are given a prescription:

1. Does my age affect the dose of my medication?

2. When and how often should I take the medicine?

3. How long before the medicine starts working?

4. How should I take the medicine—before, during, or after meals? In the morning or at bedtime?

5. What are the side effects of this medication?

6. Are there any restrictions on what I can do—like drive a car—when I am taking the medicine?

7. How will I know if the medicine is working?

8. Does this interact with other medicines I am taking?

9. Do over-the-counter medicines, vitamins, or supplements interfere or effect the medication?

10. Is there a generic version of this medication that works just as well?

them. There's the rash that sometimes develops when a patient takes one of the gout medicines or the rash that a child might develop after taking the antibiotics ampicillin or amoxicillin for what's often a viral illness. Some medicines used for the treatment of sexually transmitted diseases or for

Kevin's Comments

When I was a resident, I was fortunate enough to have an older doctor as one of my teachers. I was telling him about one of my patients who had been put on an older blood pressure medicine for months by one of my fellow residents. It was known to produce some side effects in men that affected sexual functioning. There weren't as many blood pressure medicine choices back then, so we had to use some of these medicines as first-line drugs. He told me to be very specific when I asked my patient about his side effects, especially since this man was a country farmer.

I went in to see the patient and asked my standard first question, "How are you doing on that blood pressure medicine I gave you last week?" He told me that he was doing fine and that he felt a little better. I then decided to be brave and ask him about his sexual functioning. "Are you having any sexual problems?" He told me that it did affect his "nature" a bit. At first, I had no idea what he was talking about, but it finally dawned on me. I really got nervous before I got up the courage to ask him the next question. "Are you having problems getting your manhood up anymore?" A big smile crossed the man's face and he proceeded to tell me that this was exactly the problem, but that no one had ever asked him about it before. He hated it, but never knew that the medicine could be the cause.

I took him off the medicine and put him on another that was not known to cause those problems. I saw him again in two weeks and he was proud to tell me that he was a new man.

vaginal infections can cause severe nausea and vomiting if alcohol is taken when the drug is in your system. Other medicines can produce a severe skin reaction when a person goes out in the sun. Other reactions are more personal and sometimes are difficult for patients to talk about unless questioned specifically.

Many of the antidepressants in the class of Zoloft and Prozac can cause a decrease in libido in both men and women or a change in orgasms. Doctors need to ask about these problems before beginning the medicines and after placing patients on them. Most people will not volunteer this kind of information or discuss these very personal issues unless asked specifically. If you don't help your doctor with this information, he or she won't know to make the necessary changes. What can you do to help? Again, tell your doctor about any changes in your body after you've begun taking a medicine.

THE DANGERS OF NEW DRUGS: TAKING UNNECESSARY RISKS

Dr. Sidney Wolfe, director of the nonprofit Public Citizen Health Research Group, coauthored a study that appeared in the *Journal of the American Medical Association*. This study showed that of 548 new drugs approved by the FDA from 1975 through 1999, slightly greater than 10 percent of them were withdrawn from the market or were required to have a special danger warning put on them because of specific safety concerns. Half of the drug withdrawals occurred within two years of a drug's debut. Half of the danger or "black box" warnings in the *Physician's Desk Reference* were added less than seven years after a drug was approved. What this suggests to patients is that older drugs, those on the market for at least seven years, might be better choices in many instances. There are two primary reasons why it takes so long for many of the dangerous side effects to show up. One, there are usually not enough patients tested before a drug comes to market; and two, very few of the side effects are voluntarily reported to Medwatch, the FDA's system for collecting adverse drug effect data. What should you do? Ask your doctor if the drug he is prescribing is new, and if so, are there safer alternatives that have fewer side effects that have been on the market longer.

THE HEALTH CARE TEAM MEMBER THAT COULD SAVE YOUR LIFE: YOUR PHARMACIST

We believe that you should choose your pharmacist and your pharmacy with as much care and consideration as you choose your physician. Christine's father is a pharmacist and she had a front-row seat watching the critical role that a pharmacist plays in a patient's overall health. You want to have all of the records about all of your medications in the hands of one pharmacist, who knows you, in one pharmacy. This was easier to do when your local pharmacy was a privately owned business with a single pharmacist who knew you and your family on a first-name basis.

Today, when you go to a pharmacy, it is often in a large-chain drugstore or supermarket. The pharmacist not only does not know you on a first-name basis, she can't even see you because you are so far removed from her line of vision. Often, the only people you get to see are pharmacy assistants or the cashier who makes you sign the insurance slip or the confirmation that you have been told about how the prescription you are taking works. Many of us have come to accept this new, almost nonexistent relationship with our pharmacists. We shouldn't. If you care about your health, you need to have as close a personal relationship with your pharmacist as you do with each of the doctors on your health care team. It's important to find a pharmacist who blends the high-technology capabilities of today with the personal attention that you remember from pharmacists of the past. It is possible to get the best of both worlds. You just need to know what to look for and what to ask for.

Your pharmacist isn't only there to dispense your medications. He can play a critical role in protecting your health. Pharmacists can help you by preventing unexpected side effects as well as life-threatening drug interactions. But the only way that they can help you is if you give them all of the vital information that they need . . . and if you get involved.

Most of us know more about how to order a bottle of wine at a restaurant or the features of our new cell phone than we do about the medications, prescription and over-the-counter, that we take each day. When patients are filling out their medical histories and have not brought their medications with them, the vast majority cannot pronounce or spell the name of the drugs they are taking or even tell us what color and shape they are, much less tell us the dosage. This is not a good thing. At the very minimum, knowing how to pronounce the name of your medicine and what it looks like could prevent a whole lot of dangerous mistakes and side effects down the road.

Here's what doctors—including one who is the daughter of a pharmacist—know, and you should too about developing the best possible relationship with your pharmacist:

1. You should get to know your pharmacist and your pharmacist should take the time to know everything that you and your physician can share about any current conditions that you are being treated for.

2. Your pharmacist should be informed of your medical history, in as much detail as possible. This would include, but not be limited to:

   - Your current symptoms/conditions being treated
   - Any previous illnesses that you have been treated for, including dates
   - Any previous operations that you have had, including outpatient procedures like oral surgery
   - Illnesses that run in your family
   - All medications (including over-the-counter medications, herbal medicines, and vitamin supplements) that you are taking
   - Any allergies to medications or foods that you might have
   - If you are trying to lose weight, any special diet that you are on

■ If you are pregnant, breast-feeding, or planning to become pregnant

3. Your pharmacist should be willing not only to answer your questions personally, but to call your physician or dentist on your behalf if need be.

4. Your pharmacist can serve as your advocate to help you with insurance coverage. Some insurance companies will only reimburse you for certain drugs made by certain companies. Your pharmacist can tell you which of your prescription medications will be covered by your insurance plan. A good personal relationship with your pharmacist can save you money.

5. You should choose a pharmacist whom you can talk to in a private area without other people having the ability to hear you. If you have to talk about your personal health issues in a public setting while your neighbors are waiting in line along with you, you are unlikely to be as forthright as you need to be. And if you aren't, your pharmacist won't be able to give you the very best care.

6. You should choose a pharmacist whom you can reach easily in an emergency.

7. To get the most of your relationship with your pharmacist, you should get all of your medications, both prescription and over-the-counter, from the same pharmacy.

There is a publication called the *PDR* or *Physician's Desk Reference* that lists all currently available prescription medications along with information about them, including how to prescribe, side effects, reproductive safety, toxicology, and common interactions or safety tips. There are long lists of common side effects, even if seen only in 1 percent of patients. Because there are about seventeen thousand medicines, physicians cannot possibly know all of them or their side effects. That's why it's imperative that you as a patient research and know about these possible effects. One great way to do this is to take advantage of the services that many pharmacies provide. Almost all of them offer counseling to persons receiving prescriptions. This teaches patients about their medicines, especially what to expect in the way of side effects, how to take them safely, and what other medicines, vitamins, or supplements might react with them. Take advantage of this. Why take a chance when drug interactions are so easy to prevent?

PHARMACOGENOMICS: PERSONALIZED MEDICINE FOR EVERYONE?

Doctors write thousands of prescriptions every day, but as noted earlier, they are almost flying blind when it comes to knowing how a specific patient will react to a medicine. A doctor can make a brilliant diagnosis and prescribe an appropriate medication. The problem is, the doctor can't be sure if the drug will have any beneficial effect, or will trigger some horrible side effect. The hope for the future is that a doctor could perform a genetic scan of a patient's DNA, determine if the drug she wants to prescribe will work, and then personalize the medicine. "Personalizing" drug treatment is a dream for the future and will take much of the guesswork—and the worry—out of prescribing medicines. This dream is what pharmacogenomics is all about.

Pharmacogenomics is the study of genetic factors responsible for drug response in patients. Each one of us metabolizes or processes a drug differently, based upon our unique genetic makeup. Just as our genes determine the color of our eyes and hair, so does our genetic composition determine how drugs interact with our body.

Because of the differences in our genetic makeup, some people will metabolize a drug quickly while others break it down more slowly. On average, one in ten people will be predisposed to an adverse drug reaction because they do not process a drug as expected by their doctor. If a patient is a poor metabolizer of a medicine, then the drug will stay in her system longer and she will need a lower dose. By giving a patient with slow metabolism a normal dose a doctor is increasing the risk of her developing toxic side effects. On the other hand, a person who metabolizes a drug more quickly will require a higher dose before a therapeutic effect can be seen. If doctors knew that a patient was, in fact, a high metabolizer, they would feel safer trying a higher-than-normal dose of a medicine if a patient didn't appear to experience any benefit from a usual dose. If the doctor had no knowledge of the person's metabolism, he would not be likely to try higher doses because they significantly increase the risk of adverse side effects.

DRUG DEVELOPMENT AND PHARMACOGENOMICS

For every drug eventually reaching the marketplace, there are five or six others that fail to make it because of side effects that develop in patients or a failure of the drug to show expected benefits. This trial-and-error process is extremely slow, frustrating, risky, and very expensive. As a result, pharmaceutical companies are always looking for ways to streamline the drug discovery process.

Pharmacogenomics gives pharmaceutical companies the ability to use genetic information to identify the patients most likely to respond positively to a particular drug and those who will develop side effects. Drug therapy becomes targeted to very specific patient populations. Here's a very real practical example: There are a class of drugs called "statins" that lower cholesterol. There are a number of drugs within this group and all work to lower LDL or "bad" cholesterol and have a minimal effect on raising HDL or "good" cholesterol. Ideally, it would be nice to find patients who would profit from both lowering the bad and raising the good. A new study identifies a group of patients who share a common genetic trait that allows them to receive this double benefit from these cholesterol-lowering drugs.

Similarly, it was believed for years that hormone replacement therapy after menopause would reduce women's risk of developing heart disease by maintaining levels of the body's estrogen. Two recent studies have not supported this theory and, in fact, demonstrate that HRT increases the risk of heart disease and certain cancers. An additional analysis of one of these studies looked for genetic variations in the women taking estrogen or a combination estrogen-progestin drug and found one particular genetic combination in 19 percent of women who had the biggest increases in HDL or good cholesterol levels. It was an increase that was twice as much as that of patients who didn't have the genetic variation. The researchers stated that in other studies, this increase would have been associated with around a 30 percent decrease in heart attacks or other cardiovascular events. This is just another indication of how important knowledge of our genetic makeup will be in the future.

Pharmaceutical companies worry that their profits will decrease from pharmacogenomically derived drug development because the patient population utilizing a drug will be smaller. This may be true but companies may actually gain more of a market share in a particular drug by reducing side effects in selected patients. Patients and physicians will be less worried about adverse side effects and use that particular drug even more.

The primary impact that pharmacogenomics can have on drug development is in determining early why a drug can have bad side effects on one group of people while working well on the majority. Some drugs that have failed general drug trials may, in fact, be extremely beneficial in the right patient population that has been genetically defined. By knowing this, drug companies can test a drug using only those people likely to respond favorably. This means fewer numbers of patients will need to be studied, and this lower drug development costs and increases the likelihood of newer, more focused drugs coming to market sooner.

Another big piece of the puzzle that pharmacogenomic companies are working on right now is the diagnostic tests that will be used to identify those who should use a particular drug and which particular drug to use in those patients. Pharmacogenomic companies are working to provide genetic testing kits that are simple and easy to use so that patients can take their own individual genetic data with them to their doctors. Once doctors know what drugs work best with a particular genetic code, they can better prescribe for their patients. Some pharmacogenomic companies believe that they will soon be able to prevent serious adverse drug reactions for 80 percent of all drugs currently on the market. The hope for the very near future is that pharmacogenomics will allow doctors to identify patients more likely to respond favorably to therapy or those with a greater chance of developing an adverse reaction to a drug therapy. In some cases, the future is now.

DIRECT-TO-CONSUMER ADVERTISING (DTC): ARE PHARMACEUTICAL MANUFACTURERS TRYING TO PRESCRIBE YOUR TREATMENT?

Spending for direct-to-consumer advertising of drugs totaled $2.8 billion in 2001. This was up 750 percent from 1997. Prescription drug advertisers are now among the top twenty spenders among TV advertisers. Do you really think that the pharmaceutical companies would spend all this money if DTC advertising wasn't working? Hardly. These ads are a very savvy bet on the part of pharmaceutical companies that by appealing directly to consumers, a demand can be created that is hard for physicians to counter. In fact, a 1997 survey of family physicians found this to be true: 71% believed DTC ads pressure doctors into prescribing drugs that they normally wouldn't prescribe.

In the old days of drug marketing, pharmaceutical companies focused their efforts on physicians. They sponsored conferences, advertised in medical journals, and sent hordes of pharmaceutical representatives to physician's offices, where they offered many goodies as well as samples of various drugs. Much of this persists, but in 1997, when the FDA relaxed the rules on direct-to-consumer advertising of pharmaceuticals, a revolution in drug advertising began. This new DTC approach has been so successful that according to a Kaiser Family Foundation study, 30 percent of those surveyed asked their physician about a drug they saw advertised for their condition.

Last year, prescription drug sales soared to $400 billion worldwide, with about half of that happening in the biggest market—the United States. A study by the National Institute of Health Care Management found that the fifty most heavily advertised drugs accounted for almost half of the $21 billion increase in drug sales in 1999 and 2000.

Studies by the FDA and the Kaiser Foundation show that when patients request a specific drug, doctors prescribe it 44 percent to 69 percent of the time. Generally, the drugs advertised in DTC ads are brand-name medications that are more expensive than other available medications that can treat the same problem and, in many cases, don't work better than many cheaper alternatives (brand-name anti-inflammatories are a good example of this). Because doctors are so pushed for time during office hours, they often feel that it's easier to write the prescription requested than to take the time to explain why it might not be needed at a particular time or why a less costly alternative is just as good. Maintaining patient satisfaction is another reason doctors often cite why they feel compelled to write prescriptions that result from DTC advertising. These might not be good reasons, but they're reality.

Christine's Comments

My father is still a practicing pharmacist in an upper-middle-class suburb of Los Angeles. Several times a day, patients come in and ask him for drugs that they have seen advertised on television. He tells them that they are prescription medications and that they need to go to their doctor, get an examination, and see if they actually need the allergy medication or the antidepressant they're asking about. The next patient request? They ask my father to call their physician and see if the doctor will just call in a prescription for the medication that they want, bypassing the consultation and office visit. The scary statistic? My father says that more often than not, the doctor's office tells him to fill the prescription—without the doctor seeing the patient. Does direct-to-consumer advertising work? You bet it does.

Prescribing these DTC medications unnecessarily drives up health care costs for everyone. It's just one more reason why the drug cost portion of business health plans increased 19.8 percent from 2000 to 2001.

Lawmakers are currently considering whether or not to tighten rules governing advertising and labeling for prescription drugs, especially when it comes to advertising drugs for uses for which they haven't yet been approved. Of course, the drug industry and advertisers oppose any changes to current rules, as it would significantly limit their ability to drive consumers to their doctor's offices. It will be interesting to see how this plays out, but we'll put our money on the lobbying efforts of big business once again.

Don't get us wrong, there are some benefits to this advertising. Patients are alerted to certain conditions that need treatment. For instance, people who could benefit from cholesterol-lowering drugs and who learn of their existence through the DTC ads are potentially helped by these ads.

It would help if physicians and/or medical organizations took the lead in educating patients about some of the false and misleading claims made in DTC ads. A big part of the problem is that many patients believe that DTC advertising is regulated by the FDA and permitted only for drugs that are safe and effective. That couldn't be further from the truth. The FDA doesn't have the resources to adequately monitor DTC advertising, so it's up to consumers to be wary and use their common sense. Like any other advertisements, these DTC ads are there to sell a product. It's as simple as that. You have to look past the hype and get to the underlying facts.

Would you buy a car based on a movie star's suggestion without checking out the facts? I hope not, but that's what pharmaceutical companies hope you'll do when it comes to prescription drugs. Because traditional advertising has lost much of its credibility, ad agencies are looking for more subtle approaches. If you watch television, you now get the added bonus of hearing about how a new medication changed a celebrity's life in a barrage of commercials designed to capture your attention.

Many companies are relying on celebrities, trendsetters, or ordinary consumers in an effort to move beyond the traditional television commercial or magazine ad—without an overt hint of payment for their services. In 2002, the *New York Times* revealed that celebrities—or their favorite charities— were receiving payments from drug companies to talk up their products on various talk shows and during interviews with the press. Rob Lowe, Larry King, and Montel Williams have all received compensation from health care companies. Kathleen Turner directed those watching one of her television appearances to a Web site for a rheumatoid arthritis drug. Actress Lauren Bacall made a controversial appearance on NBC's *Today* show in which she plugged a product, but failed to disclose that she was being paid for doing so.

Drug companies can avoid federal drug advertising regulations by hiring these celebrities because the companies say they are using them to raise awareness about a disease. According to the regulations, all prescription drug ads must state the drug's adverse effects and not hype its effectiveness. As long as celebrities don't mention a drug by name, the FDA considers what they do to be educational, but television networks are concerned. CNN has since announced that they will disclose all financial ties during broadcasts if a celebrity mentions a drug. The other three major networks are expected to do the same. What's our message to you? Take what you hear with a grain of healthy skepticism and do your own research before asking for any drug.

Physicians need to be armed with the facts when confronted with patient requests. They need to use the most efficacious drug based on clinical evidence. It can't be all about cost, but each drug must be tailored to a specific patient's needs. Oftentimes, the generic version of a drug works just as well as a brand name, so why pay more? When your physician wants to prescribe a drug, ask if a generic version is available or a cheaper drug that is just as beneficial. The cost of drugs in health plans all over the country has risen so rapidly that many health benefit plans are now breaking the drug benefit out separately and requiring a different premium or making employees pay more out-of-pocket costs. It's another reason why we want to arm you with the facts. We believe that information and education enable you to make the best decision for you and your family.

THE PROBLEM OF ANTIBIOTIC RESISTANCE

Prior to the development of antibiotics in the 1940s, infectious diseases were the leading cause of mortality and morbidity. It's said that more soldiers died of infected wounds (many of the infections were a result of surgery) than were killed in battle. Since their introduction, antibiotics have been the primary treatment for bacterial infections and have often been called miracle drugs. Millions of lives have been saved thanks to their use.

Unfortunately, just as many believed the battle of "drugs against bugs" was being won, bacterial organisms that were resistant to some of these antibiotics began to develop. Throughout the 1980s, the problem continued to grow even though more and more antibiotics were coming on the market. Today, one of the major problems facing medicine is the emergence of drug-resistant microorganisms or bacteria—thanks mostly to the overuse of antibiotics. A few studies have reported that more than 50 percent of patients diagnosed with common colds receive antibiotics, even though they are of no benefit in the treatment of viral illnesses. National medical organizations, including the Infectious Disease Society of America (IDSA), have identified antibiotic resistance as a major concern. Today, as a result, there are no effective therapies for some patients in hospitals. Here are a few more examples:

- About 50 percent of the most common bacteria causing diarrhea are resistant to a relatively new class of antibiotics.

- About one-third of the germs responsible for the most common form of pneumonia are now resistant to many antibiotics on the market today.

- *Staphylococcus aureus* is one of the most prevalent types of bacteria, but now in hospitals, more than half of the infections related to it

> **20 to 50 percent of antibiotic prescriptions written by doctors may be unnecessary**

are resistant to commonly used antistaph drugs. In nursing homes, the number goes up to 71 percent.

This resistance was originally confined to hospitals, but now is emerging as a community problem. Why is this happening and what can be done about it?

It's clear that antibiotic resistance is directly proportional to the volume of antibiotic consumption. The fewer antibiotics used, the less resistance develops. Studies have indicated that 20 to 50 percent of antibiotic prescriptions written by doctors may be unnecessary. Of 150 million antibiotic prescriptions written each year for patients outside of hospitals, about a third—50 million—are unnecessary, according to the Centers of Disease Control and Prevention (CDC).

Why is this happening? Many people demand antibiotics when they have a cold, even though colds are caused by viruses, and antibiotics work only against bacteria, not against viruses. Some reasons that doctors too often and too readily prescribe antibiotics include inadequate time to explain to patients (or parents) why antibiotics are unnecessary, misdiagnosis of nonbacterial infections, and the desire to keep good patient relationships. Other concerns include fear of litigation, pressure to substitute therapy for expensive diagnostic tests, misleading advertising by drug companies, and productivity incentives in managed care organizations.

Another factor contributing to this increase in antimicrobial resistance is the widespread use of antibiotics in animals and agriculture to prevent disease and aid growth. Nearly half of the antibiotics administered in the United States are used in animals. Yet another possible cause for the increase in resistance is the overuse of antibacterial substances in commonly used consumer products: soaps, lotions, cleaning products, bedding, and toothbrushes. We are vigorously destroying the disease-causing organisms, but at the same time we are also wiping out the beneficial bugs that help keep the disease-causing bacteria in check.

What can be done to slow the increasing rate of resistance? The answer requires action on the part of both physicians and patients. Physicians should not accommodate patient requests for unneeded antibiotics, should use targeted antibiotics rather than broad-spectrum medicines, should educate patients about the proper use of antibiotics, not prescribe them for viral illnesses, and should use evidence-based guidelines for prescribing them.

Sore throats are the second-most-common symptomatic reason for seeking medical care in the United States. Most sore throats are due to upper respiratory tract viruses. The only cause of sore throat deserving treatment with an antibiotic is a streptococcus bacterial infection. Only between 15 and 36 percent of children cultured have the infection, and it's found in only 5 to 17 percent of adults. Why then are 76 percent of adults diagnosed with sore throat treated with antibiotics? And when they are so treated, why are they treated with the wrong antibiotic? A recent survey in *JAMA* (September 2001) found that nonrecommended antibiotics were used in the treatment of sore throats 68 percent of the time. Instead of using penicillin or erythromycin (for penicillin-allergic patients), patients were given broad-spectrum, powerful antibiotics like Zithromax or Biaxin. Not only is this practice much more costly, but it also greatly increases the likelihood of resistance in the future.

Middle ear infections in children are another major problem area with respect to antibiotics. Otitis media (middle ear infection) is the most common diagnosis in children for which antibiotics are prescribed; it occurs when viral or bacterial organisms spread from the nose to the middle ear. Three main bacteria cause most of these infections, but they are becoming increasingly resistant to treatment because doctors are using too many broad-spectrum antibiotics.

According to a March 2003 report that appeared in the *Annals of Internal Medicine,* researchers found that doctors are more likely to use more expensive, broad-spectrum antibiotics instead of those with a narrower, more focused range. During the past ten years, the use of such nonspecific antibiotics doubled in both adults and children. According to the report, as of 1999, nearly half of antibiotics prescribed to adults and 40 percent of those prescribed to children were of the broad-spectrum variety.

Broad-spectrum antibiotics—such as azithromycin (Zithromax), clarithromycin (Biaxin), and the quinolones (Cipro and Floxin)—are effective against certain types of bacteria that cannot be treated by narrow-spectrum, more specific antibiotics. However, the types of bacteria broad-spectrum antibiotics were originally designed to combat are the ones that most often cause problems in severe, complicated infections. They are highly unlikely to be responsible for the more common respiratory tract infections that cause most of us to see our doctors. The bottom line for your pocketbook: In 2003 dollars, the retail cost is about eighty dollars for a week's worth of one of the newest broad-spectrum antibiotic compared to about fifteen dollars for a week's worth of penicillin or erythromycin. We say that if a narrow-spectrum drug will do the job, pocket the sixty-five-dollar difference and go out to dinner to celebrate your recovery and the return of your appetite.

The concern over antibiotic resistance is so great that the CDC and the American Academy of Pediatrics developed programs in 1998 to promote the appropriate and judicious use of these medications in children. Parents can help with this. Antibiotics should not be used for illnesses likely to be caused by viruses, such as colds and bronchitis, and should not be asked for

Oral Contraceptives and Antibiotics

One of the things that doctors often forget to mention to their female patients who take oral contraceptives, is that the antibiotics that they have prescribed for them could potentially interfere with the effectiveness of their oral contraceptives, and that for the rest of that cycle, they should use a back-up method of birth control.

So remember, even if your doctor or nurse does not mention it, if you are taking oral contraceptives and are taking antibiotics, always use a back-up method of contraception.

if the signs and symptoms that a patient has are probably associated with respiratory viruses, such as a runny nose and cough. Doctors often take their cue from patients, so don't insist on antibiotics in these situations, and question your doctor if she offers you one.

The most important thing that patients can do is not to demand antibiotics for every illness and insist that your doctor prescribe them only when an illness is bacterial in cause. In the latter case, ask for the medication most specific for that particular infection. If the illness is viral, learn how to treat the symptoms, and then give the body's own defense mechanisms time to cure it. The University of Arkansas for Medical Sciences conducted a study in which they produced an eight-minute video for patients that explained why antibiotics are not needed for a cold. Nine months after viewing this tape, 93 percent of patients in the study knew that antibiotics should only be used rarely, while only 71 percent of patients who did not view the tape knew this fact. Doctors at the University of Arkansas were educated at the same time about proper antibiotic use. As a result, antibiotic use in the practice dropped by about one-third.

Unless doctors and patients learn to use drugs more carefully, the bugs will continually outsmart the drugs. Education for both doctors and patients is the key.

WHAT DOCTORS KNOW ABOUT
Antibiotics . . . And You Should Too

1. The common cold does not require an antibiotic.

2. Avoid using antibiotics for upper respiratory infections (URIs) unless they are true bacterial infections (80 percent of URIs are viral, not bacterial).

3. Use narrow-spectrum antibiotics specifically indicated for a particular disease.

4. Wait at least forty-eight to seventy-two hours after taking an antibiotic before asking for a change because it takes that long for all antibiotics to begin to work.

MEDICINE MISTAKES DOCTORS
KNOW NOT TO MAKE

Medicines can be good for you ... or bad for you. Paracelsus, the great ancient Greek physician, stated that the only difference between a poison and a medicine was the dose. The beneficial effect of a drug depends not only on the dosage, but on the way the individual patient handles it. There are a number of simple things that doctors know about medications that you should too.

1. **Don't have prescriptions filled at various pharmacies.** Surveys suggest that almost 30 percent of Americans shop at several different pharmacies. The big advantage you gain by going to one pharmacy is that the pharmacist has a record of all your medicines and the dose prescribed. This is extremely important because it allows the pharmacist to spot potential drug interactions. For instance, if you take the antibiotic erythromycin with certain decongestants, you can develop a fatal heart arrhythmia.

2. **Don't stop your medicines when you start to feel better ... unless you talk to your doctor.** Stopping medicines when you begin to feel better is potentially dangerous in both the short term and long term depending on the medicine: If you stop an antibiotic before taking the full course, not all the bugs may be killed; you risk falling ill with the same infection and may also create bacterial resistance. Likewise, if you are taking steroid medicines and stop them abruptly, it can cause create serious hormonal problems. There are amazing new drugs that lower cholesterol and can prevent heart attacks. But they

can't help you if you don't take them. Studies show that 15 to 50 percent of patients who were prescribed cholesterol-lowering drugs weren't taking them a year later. Our suggestion: Drop something else off of your to-do list; leave "taking my medicine" on.

3. **Consider low-dose or no-dose.** Definitely discuss the option of the lowest possible dose of a medication that your doctor would consider to be effective. Also, keep an open mind about *no*-dose alternatives like exercise and weight loss.

4. **Double-check the medicines that you get from your pharmacist.** Pharmacists are only human and they can make mistakes (especially if they are trying to read the chicken scratchings that many doctors try to pass off as writing). Check the name of the medicine, the dose, and the number that the doctor wrote for you to make sure you are getting what your doctor prescribed.

5. **Don't give your medicines to other people (and don't take their meds either).** It's just common sense, but you won't believe how often we have heard this story from people. How do you know whether a medicine is the right one for you? Are you sure that what someone is giving you is really what they say it is? It's too easy to have a reaction to another drug, especially if it interacts with something you are already taking. You won't have enough of the drug to do you any real good anyway, so why take it? Also, suppose you took someone else's medicine, which contained a narcotic, and then you were drug-tested at work. You'd find yourself busted for no good reason.

6. **Be careful when you try to save money with drugs.** Since a twenty-milligram tablet costs as much as a ten-milligram tablet on most insurance plans, some people try to save some money by asking for a prescription for the larger pills and splitting them in half. Always ask your pharmacist if it is safe to split a pill. It was reported in a recent study that Lipitor, Viagra, and nine other drugs could be safely split in half. This is pretty easy to do when the pills are notched in the

middle. If the pill does not have that notching, you can buy a pill-cutter for around five dollars. However, you must never try to cut capsules, pills that are enteric-coated (to prevent stomach upset), or extended-release medications.

7. **Don't store your medicines in cabinets where children can reach them or in the bathroom medicine cabinet.** Many accidental poisonings occur because children reach medicines that are *not* in locked or childproof cabinets. Children tend to put anything into their mouths if possible. Don't take a chance. Also, moisture can get into medicines left in bathrooms, causing them to break down.

8. **Take most medicines on an empty stomach.** There are certain medicines that should not be taken on an empty stomach, but your pharmacist will tell you this by placing a label on the container. It's also not a good idea to take your medicines with carbonated beverages or hot liquids, as these can break down a pill before it is absorbed in the best area of your intestine.

9. **Ask your pharmacist about your medicines; don't rely on your doctor.** We know this might sound a bit crazy, but the doctor writing your prescription may not be aware of all the medicines you are taking and of certain drug interactions. Doctors do not spend a great deal of time learning about drug interactions in their training. Pharmacists learn about the medications they dispense and know much more than the average physician about side effects and drug interactions. Pharmacists have called us on numerous occasions to ensure that we understood certain issues about a medication we had just prescribed. We always appreciated this, and in most instances obtained information that we had not been aware of.

OVER-THE-COUNTER (OTC) MEDICATIONS

Market survey data indicates that more than 70 percent of American adults and 50 percent of American children take nonprescription, over-the-counter (OTC) medicines in any given month. OTC medications provide prompt, low-cost relief for certain symptoms. More than 100,000 OTC products were available to consumers in 2002, but a relatively small number of active ingredients were used in these medications.

Before a medication can be marketed without a prescription, the FDA requires that an OTC meet the following standards:

- The medication must possess a low risk of side effects at the effective dose level.

- Patients must be able to self-diagnose their symptoms and select an appropriate treatment.

- The product labeling must be easy to read and easy to understand and must include indications, contraindications, and directions for use.

The majority of OTC products can be put into one of the following classifications: pain relievers, antihistamines, decongestants, and cough medications.

Side Effects and OTCs

OTC medications are generally very safe, and when used by most healthy adults, there is an almost complete absence of serious side effects. But don't forget: OTCs are drugs and are not risk free. Certain groups of patients are at increased risk of injury from OTC medicines: the young, the elderly, those with poor kidney function, and persons taking multiple medications.

Pharmacists are especially concerned about the way that consumers medicate themselves with over-the-counter drugs, and a recent survey commissioned by the National Council on Patient Education and Information backed them up. One-third of consumers say that they take more than the recommended dose of a nonprescription medicine, believing that more is better. A third also say that they are likely to combine nonprescription medicines when they have multiple symptoms, like a sore throat and a headache. This practice increases the risk that a patient is taking more than one OTC product at a time that contains the same active ingredient.

Over-the-Counter Pain Relievers

When many Americans were growing up, if they had a headache or any ache or pain, they went to the medicine chest and took aspirin. Today, if you go to your local supermarket or drugstore to find something for your headache, you'll probably be faced with over a hundred different over-the-counter choices. You'll see a big difference in packaging and promises, but pretty much all of the over-the-counter, nonprescription pain relievers contain one of the following: aspirin, ibuprofen, acetaminophen, naproxen sodium, or ketoprofen. Not needing a prescription makes these medications easy to obtain, but using them safely may not be as simple. The biggest problem: Most of us have no idea that there could be *any* risks associated with an over-the-counter medication.

Which of the hundred options is right for you? All over-the-counter pain relievers can relieve minor pains that are associated with headaches, muscle aches, backaches, menstrual cramps, arthritis, toothaches, and colds and flu. Nonsteroidal anti-inflammatory drugs (NSAIDS)—which include aspirin and ibuprofen (i.e., Motrin and Advil)—do double duty. They reduce inflammation while they relieve pain. This is key because controlling your inflammation can go a long way toward reducing your pain. But certain patients experience side effects with these pain relievers: dizziness, drowsiness, headaches, gastrointestinal distress, and even high blood pressure. Acetaminophen only relieves pain . . . it can't reduce inflammation.

But with fewer side effects, it is a good option if you can't afford the side effect associated with NSAIDS.

OTC pain relievers like aspirin and the NSAIDS like ibuprofen and naproxen (Advil, Aleve, etc.) increase the risk of gastrointestinal bleeding that is dose related. The more you take, the greater the risk of GI bleeding. Combining the two drugs significantly increases the risk of bleeding. Using alcohol along with these medicines (even as little as one drink per week), also increases the risk of bleeding.

A large number of OTC and prescription medications contain acetaminophen as well as pain relievers. These include: cold remedies, headache medications, and sleeping aids. It is important to calculate your overall daily exposure to acetaminophen from all sources. Why is this important? Too much acetaminophen can lead to kidney and liver damage, and in large enough doses, even death. If you take acetaminophen drugs like Tylenol regularly, you should avoid alcohol to reduce the risk of serious damage to your liver.

Many consumers have the misperception that OTCs are not "real" medicines, so they don't report their use to their doctors. They also aren't as careful about understanding the ingredients in the different drugs or calculating and measuring the proper dose. Surveys have proven that patients knowingly use OTC medications in a manner that is inconsistent with product labeling. Patients tend to think of brand-name OTCs and do not think of active ingredients in the medication. It's easy to take more of a certain ingredient than is recommended because many OTCs have two to five active ingredients.

WHAT DOCTORS KNOW ABOUT
Taking OTC Pain Relievers Safely . . . And You Should Too

1. **Talk to Your Pharmacist:** To avoid dangerous drug interactions, talk with your pharmacist as well as your doctor about which over-the-counter pain reliever is best and safest for you. The best OTC pain

reliever for the person in the office next to yours is not necessarily the best one for you.

2. **Never Exceed the Recommended Dosage:** It is important not to exceed either the recommended dosage or timing, unless your doctor specifically instructs you to do so.

3. **Know Your Limitations:** You should stay away from NSAIDS (like Motrin and Advil) if you have ulcers, take blood thinners, have bleeding disorders, or are allergic to aspirin.

4. **Never Give Aspirin to Children:** Aspirin has been linked to Reye's syndrome, which is a potentially fatal swelling of brain tissue in children and in teenagers.

5. **OTC Pain Meds and Alcohol Do Not Mix:** Mixing alcohol with NSAIDS like aspirin and ibuprofen can lead to stomach upset and bleeding. If you combine too-high doses of acetaminophen with alcohol, you can end up with serious damage to your liver.

6. **Milk and Food DO Mix with OTC Pain Relievers:** You can minimize any possible stomach upset by not taking these OTC pain relievers on an empty stomach.

OTC Weight Loss Products: Do They Really Work?

Each day, millions of Americans struggle to look like the thin and appealing stars that they see on television and in magazines. Two-thirds of Americans are either overweight or obese. Individuals who are obese and need to lose a hundred pounds or more, and people who want to lose ten pounds to look better at their high school reunion, turn to diet pills. And everyone is looking for the same solution: an easy one. The result? A multibillion-dollar diet supplement industry that promises us a miracle in a pill—a perfect body and a new life all in a matter of weeks.

But, as we all know, losing weight requires burning more calories than we take in. It's a simple math equation: The calories that we burn have to be greater than the calories we take in when we eat each day. As depressing as it might be, if a weight loss plan sounds too good to be true, it probably is.

OTC diet aids promise to help us lose weight in two ways: by suppressing our appetites or by increasing our metabolism. However, it is important to realize that these products don't significantly influence the amount of weight you lose or your ability to keep that weight off long-term. An appetite suppressant might help some people in the short term, but unfortunately there is no substitute for exercising and developing healthy eating habits long term.

The Weight Loss Practice Survey, sponsored by the FDA and the National Heart, Lung and Blood Institute, found that 5 percent of women and 2 percent of men trying to lose weight use diet pills. The majority of these diet pills are over-the-counter (OTC) medications like Dexatrim and Acutrim and contain the active ingredient phenylpropanolamine (PPA).

According to the FDA's Office of OTC Drug Evaluation, using diet pills containing PPA will not make a big difference in the rate of weight loss. The problem with these medications is that although they can surpress your appetite initially, their effects are usually short-lived. After approximately six weeks or less, most individuals get used to the medication and the appetite suppression properties of the pills disappears. You might lose some pounds, but will probably never achieve your ideal weight and maintain your new weight long-term without permanent changes in your diet and exercise habits.

Diet pills can also be potentially dangerous. Many of these pills contain stimulants such as caffeine, guarana, and bitter orange. Some people can be sensitive to these, even without ephedra, and they may have an idiosyncratic or weird reaction leading to a rise in blood pressure, arrhythmia, restlessness, and agitation. Definitely talk to your doctor before starting OTC diet pills.

In addition to the scores of brand name weight loss products out on the market, there are three common supplements we are asked about all the time:

Chromium Picolinate: There is some research showing that this supplement helps insulin work more efficiently. It claims to improve and boost metabolism, but has never been tested or proven to be effective in scientifically sound studies in large populations.

Herbal Laxatives and Diuretics: These supplements cause you to lose water, not fat. They can lower your potassium levels and cause both heart and muscle problems. Another caution: If you use laxatives too often, your bowels can become dependent on them.

Ephedra: An ancient Chinese herbal remedy known as mahuang, this supplement is sold as a diet pill or workout enhancer. Ephedra has been linked in studies by the FDA and other organizations to hundreds of adverse effects, including hypertension, irregular heartbeat, seizure, heart attack, stroke, and death. The recent deaths of a few prominent professional athletes have been linked to ephedra use. According to a study published in the *Annals of Internal Medicine* in March 2003, 64 percent of all adverse reactions reported to poison control centers around the country that deal with herbal supplements had to do with ephedra.

WARNING: Even though many weight loss products claim to be natural or herbal, this doesn't mean they're safe. Under existing law, ephedra and other herbal supplements, unlike drugs, are not subject to premarket testing, nor are manufacturers required to report the incidence of harmful side effects. Let those who use these products beware. We would certainly not advise using them. You should not take any of these diet pills lightly. Our advice: Check with your doctor before using any diet pills—whether they are "conventional," herbal, or natural.

Supplement Health Ads— Lots of Promises But Little Performance or Benefit

We've all seen the advertisements on the Internet (mostly offering sexual enhancements for men or growth hormone to keep us young), on the back pages of magazines (you can lose twenty pounds in a month without diet or exercise), or on late-night infomercials (aging celebrities touting supplements designed to do about everything). They seem almost too good to be true . . . and trust us, they are.

Advertising of various herbal supplements and combination of vitamins and minerals is a huge business making billions for those selling them. Unfortunately, the hype and the promises found in the ads aren't matched by the actual performance. One consumer watchdog group even went so far as to say that not a single pill or potion has lived up to its promises. Pretty strong words. We don't want you throwing your money down the drain or worse, developing some bad side effect from the pills or potions you might be taking. Here are a few warning signs that things may not be on the up and up:

Five Warning Signs of Untruthful Health Ads

1. Ads that promise quick, miraculous or dramatic results—If it sounds too good to be true, then it almost always is. We'd all like to lose weight the easy way or turn back time without working at it, but that's just not possible. If these claims were true, drug companies and other major corporations would be selling the product, they wouldn't just be offered at the back of magazines or on television at 3 A.M. Don't trust these "miracle" pills, they simply don't work.

2. Ads using testimonials or anecdotes—Show us the science and don't give us stories by people that have been paid to give testimonials.

We guarantee you that they are not doing this for nothing. If the product is good, then the science will be there. Anecdotes are usually used when manufacturer's have nothing else to support their claims.

3. Consider the placement of the ad—If these ads come as spam appear in the back pages of tabloids or come in the form of infomercials that air in the wee hours of the morning be very careful. Remember that old axiom, "If you lie down with dogs, then you're going to get fleas."

4. Disclaimers in the ad using pseudo-medical terms—Be wary of the word *alternative* in ads, as it's an excuse to get away from acceptable practices. Also be very cautious when you see medical-like terms such as "detoxify" or "purify" as part of the claims.

5. Ads that use questionnaires to see if you can use the product—Have you ever seen ad in which you didn't answer "Yes" to at least one of the questions? Of course not, because they want to sell products.

Doctors know better than to trust this kind of advertising and you should too. If you see these warning signs in ads on television, in magazines and on the Internet featuring vitamins, herbs or supplements of any kind, a red flag should go up and bells and whistles should go off in your head. Don't trust there ads. If you buy most of these products, you might as well just throw or give your money away because the great majority of them won't deliver on the hype found in the ad. There's often no real science behind the products and they certainly haven't been evaluated using accept-able scientific testing methods. Our final word: Let the buyer beware.

Web sites for OTC Information

www.familydoctor.org: Patient-oriented information about OTCs from the American Academy of Family Physicians.

www.pharmacyandyou.org: The American Pharmaceutical Association provides information about various medicines including potential drug interactions.

www.fda.gov/cder/otc/ndex.htm: The U.S. Food and Drug Administration Center for Drug Evaluation and Research's over-the-counter drugs Web site provides numerous evaluations and data on OTC medications.

www.chpa-info.org: The Consumer Healthcare Products Association provides consumer information on commonly used home products.

VITAMINS, MINERALS, AND HERBAL SUPPLEMENTS

Finally, let's talk a bit about vitamins and herbal supplements, as millions of dollars are spent on them yearly and they are poorly understood. Although providing detailed information about vitamins and supplements is beyond the scope of this book (there are many excellent books devoted to them), we'd like to address a few misconceptions and provide you with some commonsense ideas before you start putting a medicine into your system. Believe us herbal supplements and vitamins are drugs and can be dangerous. Make sure to buy only from reputable companies that contain certification marks like "USP" and "NSF International." Please do not be misled by what you may have heard. If not used properly, herbal supplements and excessive vitamin intake can cause health problems.

Vitamins and Minerals

Vitamins and minerals together are called micronutrients. Your body needs them so that you can be healthy and have normal growth. Here is the key: Your body can't make micronutrients, so you have two choices: You can either get them from the foods you eat or you can get them from supplements.

There are fourteen vitamins and they fall into two categories:

1. *Fat Soluble:* Vitamins A, D, E, and K. Your body stores these in fat. Some fat-soluble vitamins, like vitamins A and D, can accumulate in your body and reach toxic levels if you take too many of them.

2. *Water Soluble:* Vitamin C, choline, biotin, and the seven B vitamins: thiamin (B_1), riboflavin (B_2), niacin (B_3), panthothenic acid (B_5), pyridoxine (B_6), folic acid/folate (B_9), and cobalamin (B_{12}). These vitamins are processed and excess amounts are passed in your urine.

There are two categories of minerals:

1. Major Minerals: These are the minerals that we need in larger amounts. They include sodium, potassium, calcium, phosphorus, magnesium, and chloride.

2. Additional Minerals: These are the minerals that we need in smaller amounts for normal growth and health: iron, fluoride, iodine, copper, chromium, selenium, zinc, manganese, molybdenium.

Except for very young children, taking a daily multivitamin is a good idea. This is especially true for preteens, teenagers, and seniors because many people in these groups do not eat balanced meals, and the lack of one or two key vitamins can cause health problems very quickly. And, there are very few risks (we can't think of any in the case of basically healthy people) associated with this practice . . . and so many rewards. Many vitamins are essential to the optimal functioning of the cells within your body. They can also improve your physical appearance and they can help put a glow in your hair and on your skin.

A recent study in the *Journal of the American Medical Association* highlights the importance of vitamins to our health. Researchers put patients on a six-month regimen of folic acid, vitamin B_{12}, and vitamin B_6 and studied whether or not this combination was useful in preventing heart disease. The researchers found that the vitamin therapy decreased by 38 percent the need for repeat angioplasties or heart bypass operations when compared to a similar group of patients who took a placebo. (One of the biggest problems with angioplasty procedures is that about one-third of patients will need another procedure within a year as a result of a recurrence of the blockage.) This is the second study to show this effect. It's believed that the treatment works by lowering levels of homocysteine, an amino acid that has been implicated in heart attacks.

When You Might Need Vitamin and Mineral Supplements

You are on a calorie-restricted diet or don't eat well: You are on a diet or if you simply don't manage your five servings of fruits and vegetables each day.

You are a postmenopausal woman: It is difficult for a lot of women to get the recommended amounts of vitamin D and calcium, both of which have been proven to help prevent osteoporosis.

You are pregnant or trying to become pregnant: If you are pregnant, you need more of certain nutrients like folic acid, calcium, and iron.

You smoke: Tobacco decreases the absorption of many important vitamins and minerals.

You take medications that interfere with nutrient absorption: If you take antibiotics, antacids, diuretics, or laxatives that interfere with your nutrient absorption, your doctor may recommend a supplement.

WHAT DOCTORS KNOW ABOUT
Vitamins and Minerals . . . And You Should Too

1. **Megadoses Can Be Dangerous:** You should choose a multivitamin-mineral supplement that has 100 percent of the RDA (recommended daily allowance) of most of the vitamins and minerals rather than megadoses of one vitamin. Most of the cases of nutrient toxicity result from people taking megadose supplements. Another risk: Megadoses can have harmful or dangerous interactions with many drugs.

2. **Pay Attention to Expiration Dates:** Vitamin and mineral supplements can lose their potency and effectiveness over time, especially if you live in a hot or a humid climate. You shouldn't buy any supplements that don't show an expiration date.

3. **Talk to Your Doctor:** Check with your doctor before taking anything other than a standard multivitamin-mineral supplement, especially if you have any health problems or are taking any medications. It's always better to be safe than sorry.

Herbal Supplements

Supplements are a whole different story. There are so many myths and misconceptions around herbs (as well as many false claims) that the average person should undertake some very serious research before taking any supplements on a regular basis. As one physician put it so well, "When you look at the data supporting health claims for supplements, in general, there's more enthusiasm than data." Here are some of the myths and misconceptions about these vegetable compounds that you need to be aware of:

Herbs are natural, so they must be safe: No matter what you've been led to believe, these are active substances that can cause problems if you're not careful. Some of today's medicines are derived from the same plants as herbal supplements, so we'd have to conclude that herbal medications are drugs. We know that certain herbs like chaparrel, kombucha tea, and comfrey shouldn't be taken by anyone. Other herbs clearly interact with medicines that you might be taking. Common herbs like ginger, garlic, and alfalfa (there are many more) can interact with anticoagulants and antiplatelet drugs and cause bleeding problems. Ginseng, St. John's wort, and chamomile can interact with antidepressant meds and cause problems. St. John's wort can lower the concentration of oral contraceptives and certain other prescription drugs. Always consult with your doctor and pharmacist before taking any herbs with medicine.

I can take an herb instead of a prescription drug: Many people would like to believe this, but most herbs have not been studied in clinical trials the way prescription drugs have so dosages, side effects, and efficacy may vary widely. Herbs may be fine in certain instances, but give us prescription drugs any day until the benefits of herbs are proven in controlled clinical trials.

It's okay to believe the claims on herbal labels and advertising: Do you believe all you see and read in TV and magazine ads? We doubt it. You certainly shouldn't when it comes to claims for herbal supplements. The advertising claims are not regulated and there is often no good scientific studies backing them up. We put many of these claims in the same category as the TV infomercials you see in the middle of the night. Do your research and regard the ads with a healthy degree of skepticism.

If a little is good, then more is better: If this statement is true for herbs, it's also time for prescription drugs or vitamins. We clearly know that there are therapeutic ranges for substances and there are toxic ranges. Sometimes the line between the two is very fine. Take too much of anything and it can cause problems. Don't exceed the recommended amount on the bottle without speaking to a reputable health professional.

Taking supplements while pregnant or breast-feeding is good: Women who would never take a prescription or OTC medication without checking with their doctor forget about herbs being potentially just as harmful to their fetus. If a drug is in a woman's system, it can affect the fetus.

The increased use of herbal remedies has led to problems in areas that might surprise you. Would you want the pilot flying your airplane using a drug that could affect his mind? Obviously not, yet a consultant to the FAA (Federal Aviation Administration) has warned physicians who specialize in examining pilots that pilots who use herbal supplements may be at risk of being incapacitated mentally or suffering other health effects. Here's another example of how using herbal supplements in certain circumstances could have deadly implications:

Anesthesiologists are reporting more complications in the surgical suite. The *Journal of the American Medical Association* reported some of these concerns in 2001, but the research may have only shown the tip of the iceberg. Ephedra, which we discussed in the section on weight loss products, may be one of the most dangerous products on the market today. Physicians should specifically ask patients which herbal or OTC medicines they are taking and to determine the dosage and length of treatment.

If you are planning to have surgery, you need to realize that herbs can have life-threatening interactions with surgical anesthesia. Most experts would recommend that any supplements be stopped at least two weeks before surgery. According to the American Society of Anesthesiologists, ginseng, golden seal, ephedra, and licorice can affect heart rate and blood pressure. The herbs that may increase your risk of bleeding during a surgical procedure are garlic, ginger, and ginkgo.

Persons taking aspirin, Plavix (super aspirin), and Coumadin to thin their blood should be warned that taking herbal supplements like garlic, ginger, or ginkgo along with these medicines might cause excessive bleeding. The herbal supplement St. John's wort can alter the body's metabolism of many drugs and should not be used if a person is taking antidepressants, digoxin (a heart medicine), theophylline (an asthma medicine), or undergoing chemotherapy.

These are just a few examples of how herbal supplements can impact your health, so it behooves all of us to be very careful about using them. There are some wonderful reference books on this subject that can be found in libraries and bookstores. We advise doing some research before mixing supplements and prescription medications because most physicians are likely to be unaware of many of the interactions.

Web sites for Herbal Information and Supplement Safety

www.mskcc.org/aboutherbs: Memorial Sloan-Kettering's fast, free consumer site with great information about supplement safety. It contains information about 140 different products and is updated regularly.

www.nal.usda.gov: USDA Food and Nutrition Web site offers a list of books, magazines, and Web sites about the science behind dietary supplements.

www.dietary-supplements.info.nih.gov: The National Institutes of Health's Office of Dietary Supplements posts safety warnings on various compounds.

Summary

Medicines need to be respected, as they all can contribute to adverse drug events. Research the medicines you have been given so that you understand the side effects. Don't wait for your doctor to ask you about them. It's your body. Know what you are putting into it. Ultimately, the responsibility for your health rests with you.

CHAPTER SEVEN

EMERGENCY MEDICINE: HOW TO GET THE BEST CARE IN THE ER

Last year, there were more than 100 million visits to emergency rooms in the United States. We doubt that there is one person in this country who has not been touched at some time, in some way, by an experience with a hospital emergency room, whether it be personally, with a family member, or with a friend. Some people have had unbelievably positive experiences, but many others have not been so fortunate. Let's look at a few.

REAL SCENES FROM THE ER

Case #1: *A young woman is brought to the ER complaining of abdominal pain. The "moonlighting" doctor on duty, who is a second-year surgical resident, believes it might be a viral gastroenteritis and misses the ectopic pregnancy in her fallopian tubes. He sends her home, but she returns a few hours later and requires emergency surgery that saves her life but leaves her sterile.*

Case #2: *A mother brings her infant child to the ER, where he is evaluated by an ER doctor whose training is in internal medicine. The child is diagnosed with a viral upper respiratory infection and the doctor misses a case of bacterial meningitis. The child is seen again the next day and immediately put on antibiotics. Unfortunately, it is too late and the child suffers brain damage.*

Case #3: *The doctor on call sees a young man who fell on his arm. He diagnoses a wrist fracture but misses the fracture in his elbow. As a result, the patient suffers permanent nerve damage in the arm, resulting in loss of motor function in his hand. The doctor was trained in medicine but had seen very few orthopedic cases.*

Case #4: *A child with active seizures is brought to the ER. Nurses try to start an IV and give some medicines, but there is no readily available pediatric equipment. The child stops breathing and again there are no child-size intubation or breathing tubes, so an airway cannot be established right away. As a result, the child vomits into her lungs and pneumonia results, causing a long and lengthy hospital stay and some mild brain damage.*

Make-believe? No, these are real scenes from real hospitals. Bad things can happen to good people in the ER. We all need to be aware that not all emergency rooms or emergency room personnel are created equal. There are some excellent health care providers, but there are others that lack the necessary training and experience to provide the proper treatment to the many people who come to ER in need of emergency care. Because of this, anyone who must go to the hospital emergency room needs to be vigilant and to exercise a certain amount of caution. Remember the old truism "Let the buyer beware." This chapter will provide you with the necessary insights to become a smart ER shopper, as well as some important tips for getting the best possible care for you and your family if you should ever find yourself in an ER.

IT'S NOT AN ER, IT JUST PLAYS ONE ON TV

ER is one of the most popular television shows in history and NBC can count on 30 million viewers tuning in to the show every week. Can you believe those numbers? Somehow or another, *ER* has struck a chord with American viewers. We think there are a few reasons for this. First, people like seeing what goes on behind the scenes of a hospital; second, most viewers have likely been to an ER or know someone who has; and third, it's a good show with good writing and strong story lines. But this television drama has given people an unrealistic view of hospital emergency rooms across the country.

It's really kind of funny. Regardless of where we meet people—on a plane, when speaking at a lecture, or at a cocktail party—when they find out that Kevin was an ER doctor for almost twenty-five years, the most frequent question that they ask is, "Is the emergency room in real life like the one on the television show?" There is such a fascination with what an ER is really like. Well, here's the answer.

First of all, life in the ER is fairly mundane, but at times the relative normalcy is interrupted by moments of sheer panic. Except on very rare occasions, no real emergency room has the constant flow of extremely sick patients that the TV show has. After all, they have to pack a lot of drama into one hour. The TV show depicts a big-city ER that is definitely busier than most ERs around the country. In all ERs, there is a definite ebb and flow to the amount of incoming patients and the severity of their problems. For the most part, Kevin worked in big-city emergency rooms, but he did put in his time in smaller, country hospital ERs as a moonlighter. There are quiet times and there are extremely busy, pull-your-hair-out, gut-wrenching times. But there are some common sounds and sights in an ER that many of you may relate to.

Picture this scene: There's a waiting room full of people who are speaking many different languages. Babies are crying. The faces of the people are anguished, worried, or bored. The ER doors open and close frequently as patients and friends constantly enter and exit. Some people are immediately whisked back to examination rooms, while others are doomed to wait for hours. Police and ambulance sirens seem constantly to break through the routine sounds of the hospital. A television is heard somewhere in the background. The sounds of people in pain or crying can be heard from time to time. It's never really quiet.

As you can see, emergency rooms can be scary places. And you should be scared. If you're in an ER, it means you or someone you care about needs immediate medical treatment, and Noah Wylie isn't going to be there to make everything turn out okay. Kevin chose to work in the ER because he wanted to help people in need, but we don't know anyone, ourselves included, who wants to be in the ER on the other side of the stethescope.

As with hospitals and doctors, all ERs are not created equal. Mistakes do happen and diagnoses are missed, as you saw from some of the previous scenarios. If you find yourself in an ER, all sorts of questions will be going through your head. Am I getting good care? How can I make sure that I'm even in the best ER to handle my problem? What can I do to help this strange doctor that I'm seeing in the ER give me the best care? What can I do after I leave to help my chances of getting better? Is this ER capable of caring for my children properly?

All these are very valid questions and concerns. We know. We've been in the same situation ourselves. We've had to bring ourselves, or our family members, to unfamiliar emergency rooms in cities where we knew nothing about the hospital, the doctors, or the ER. In our particular cases, it's definitely been a humbling experience because we are used to being in control. We had the same concerns and worries that you would have in that situation, but we had one ace in the hole. We know how emergency rooms work and how to evaluate the personnel caring for us. We know some things to do . . . and not to do. So what can you do? How can you ensure that you are doing all that you can to get the best care possible? There are definitely some things that you can do to be more in control and get the help you need. This is what this chapter is all about.

WHAT DOCTORS KNOW ABOUT
Emergency Medicine . . . And You Should Too

1. All emergency rooms are not created equal. Care can vary greatly, and it can cost you dearly if you're not careful.

2. The skill levels of emergency room doctors can vary tremendously. You have to know their background and training.

3. Nurses who work in the ER and paramedics who transport patients generally know who the best doctors are.

4. Don't go to the ER unless it's an emergency.

5. Many hospitals are not adequately equipped to take care of pediatric patients.

6. Trauma care is best done at trauma centers or tertiary care hospitals.

WHICH ER SHOULD YOU GO TO?

Let's assume that you're either in a strange city or you've not done your homework about the ERs in your area. Because you're really sick, you know you have to get to the ER by ambulance. You call 911 and ask them to send help. When the paramedics arrive, ask them what the best emergency room in the city is. Why are they the best people to ask?

Paramedics are the health care team members that staff the emergency vehicles that transport patients to the ER all the time. They know the doctors and the staff at all the hospitals. They have a great deal of inside knowledge about who's good and who's not so good. They know where they would go if they were sick. So, here's what you need to do whether you're at home or in a strange city. Ask the paramedics who come to transport you: "If you were sick, which ER would you go to?" When you hear the answer, tell them to take you to that same ER.

But what if you're in a foreign city and don't speak the language? Because of their jobs, millions of people travel both domestically and internationally on a regular basis. These "road warriors" are constantly on the go and often don't have control over where and when they are sent. Add to these frequent travelers the millions of people who travel all over the world for pleasure, and the chances of someone getting ill and needing medical attention while away from home and their regular medical care providers become quite high. Too many people take their good health for granted and forget to prepare for an emergent situation while away from home.

Many larger corporations understand that this can be a problem, so they contract with organizations such as SOS and Assist America to provide backup travel advice and medical support for their corporate travelers. These organizations will, by having you dial an 800 number, provide the name of an English-speaking doctor or the name of the best hospital in the foreign city where you find yourself. These companies will provide advice to you over the phone about your condition and can even arrange to speak to doctors in a foreign country in their native language to ensure the best possible medical care.

But, what if you're not part of a company and you're taking your elderly parents on a vacation to a foreign country. What can you do to get the best medical care in a country? There are several things that you can do ahead of time.

■ Check with AAA or the group sponsoring the trip, as they can often arrange for travel-related medical insurance.

■ Check with the U.S. embassy in that country or with the State Department before you travel.

■ Take out a personal contract with one of the organizations such as International SOS or Assist America.

HOW CAN YOU GET TO SEE THE DOCTOR MORE QUICKLY?

The average ER is no longer being used primarily as an emergency room. Instead, many people now use the ER as their primary care doctor and show up for treatment of upper respiratory infections, earaches, and other relatively minor medical problems that could be handled easily in a non-acute setting. Why is this?

The most recent data shows that 41 million people in the United States are now without medical insurance. This is more than the combined population of twenty-three states and the District of Columbia. When people don't have insurance, they don't try to see an office-based doctor but will go to free clinics or, more commonly, an ER. Many people on Medicaid or Medicare also use the ER for medical care because many doctors refuse to treat many patients in these programs because reimbursement is often less than 50 percent of their regular fees. It's a money-losing proposition for most doctors. Other populations of people frequently using emergency rooms for nonemergent problems are the homeless, the disenfranchised, and recent arrivals from foreign countries who also may not have health insurance.

So, what's this information about the uninsured have to do with your experience in the ER? It's very simple. All of these many nonemergent reasons for coming to the ER help contribute to the long waits and difficulties in being seen that we encounter in emergency rooms all over the United States. It's a fact of life, so you need to learn how to get the best care from an overworked hospital staff in this most difficult, dangerous, and busy setting.

How can you get to see the ER doctor more quickly? Hospitals use what's called a triage system to determine which patients get seen first. *Triage* is a French term, used by emergency personnel both on the scene of accidents or disasters and in emergency rooms, that means to sort out people by the severity of their medical problems. Hospitals do this to ensure that the patients who are the sickest get taken care of first.

When you come to the ER, you will likely see a triage nurse, who will assess your condition. This is not the time to downplay your symptoms. If you want to get in to see the doctor sooner, make sure to tell the triage nurse why you are in the emergency room. Persons in pain, those with emergent problems, those with injuries, and very sick children get seen first. Don't minimize your symptoms or your pain. We've heard of patients who didn't tell the ER personnel how bad they really felt, got worse, and put themselves at serious risk. If you are bringing in a sick child, tell the triage nurse why you believe he is so ill and why you are scared enough to bring him to the ER. If you don't tell the triage nurse how sick you feel, then you could be waiting for a long time.

Christine's Comments

One time when I was taken to the ER, my pulse rate was off the charts. I didn't know why it was happening at the time, but I knew that it was not a good thing. The ER was filled to capacity, but the first thing that I did was tell the nurses and the doctor that there was something wrong with my heart and that I needed immediate attention because I did not want to have a heart attack. I established that my condition was a priority and they gave me immediate attention.

When you are taken to an ER, if you are facing a potentially life-threatening situation, it is important to make your case immediately upon arriving at the ER. Do not expect that the ambulance driver or the paramedic will do the job for you. You or the person who has come with you to the ER needs to state your case—quickly and emphatically.

Fortunately for me, the doctor who took care of me that night figured out that it was acid reflux that was making my heart race. My ER story had a happy ending. But when I arrived, no one knew what was causing my problem so I had to let the ER team

know how serious my situation was especially because I didn't look as sick as I felt. It is most important to tell the doctors what your problem is and exactly how serious it might be, especially if you don't look very sick when they bring you in. The person with food poisoning might look sicker than you do, but your life might actually be at stake. Don't be a hero. Help the team in the ER save your life.

One point we can't stress enough: If you think you might be having a heart attack, let the nurse know immediately. Don't downplay your symptoms. Don't be embarrassed or afraid that you're overeating. If you say, "Well, I might have indigestion," you could have a cardiac event while you're waiting to see a doctor. Instead, be very clear about. Say, "I think I'm having a heart attack." Speaking up just might save your life.

DO THE DOCTOR AND ER SUPPORT STAFF MAKE A DIFFERENCE IN THE CARE THAT YOU GET?

You had better believe it. Receiving the correct diagnosis and getting the optimal care for both adults and children are almost completely dependent on the doctor providing the care in the emergency room. Don't kid yourself. The doctor you see in the ER is the major determining factor in the kind of care you get in the ER. If he doesn't order the right diagnostic tests, if he doesn't listen to what you're telling him, or he doesn't have the clinical experience to make the correct diagnosis, then you are in trouble. Now, before any of you readers who are ER supporting staff personnel—nurses, nursing aides, and clerical staff—jump down our throats, we know that it takes a team of people to render care from start to finish, but the doctor is the key determinant in whether or not the team does well. ERs are no different from any other service organization. They're only as good as the people providing the service. If people don't have the training, experience, equipment, or ancillary support needed, there will be problems in the kind of professional service they deliver.

Let's use an example outside of medicine to illustrate this point. In this day and age, no business can exist without computers. The bigger the business, the more computers and the bigger the network needed to support them . . . and the more things that can go wrong. If you had computer problems, you likely wouldn't go for repair to someone without experience or not skilled in the particular type of computer you own. If you did, you'd be afraid that they might make the problem worse or upset your entire system. It takes experience in a particular type of system or computer to be able to make the right assessment, to know the nuances of a computer, and to know how one type of software can affect another. For simple problems, you don't need an experienced person. It's in the unusual situation that you want and need the expert. The problem is that sometimes you don't know you have a more complex problem until you get into solving it. When you address an obvious problem, you can miss a larger one. Experience does make the difference.

Emergency room doctors and nurses are no different from the computer experts, except that their mistakes can result in severe medical complications, and can even cost someone their life. Many doctors can treat the simple problems, but in emergency situations, you want an expert who knows the most about dealing with acute medical problems. Unfortunately, not all doctors working in emergency rooms are trained in emergency medicine. Sound hard to believe? Well, you better believe it and be aware of it if you or a loved one needs to go to the ER. You need to check out the doctors who will be treating you so you can make sure you get the best possible care.

Physicians trained in emergency medicine and who become board certified in that specialty staff many emergency rooms. This is the best possible scenario for you as a patient. A physician who becomes board certified in emergency medicine has demonstrated a certain level of competency in the diagnosis of problems encountered in an emergency room setting. Such doctors are board certified by the American Board of Emergency Medicine and are members of the American College of Emergency Physicians

(ACEP). To retain that board certification, a doctor must maintain a certain level of continuing medical education in emergency-medicine-related topics every year as well as retaking her specialty exams every several years (one of only a few medical specialties to have this requirement).

In some ERs, doctors who may not be board certified in emergency medicine, but are specialists in another field, work regularly at treating patients. They choose to work in the ER because it's what they like to do. They're often called board-eligible ER doctors because of their prior work experience or their many years in the ER. The doctors who routinely work in the ER are often the physicians most able to make the correct diagnosis because this is their chosen specialty. They take pride in what they do.

Ideally, we recommend that patients look for, and should expect to find, either board-certified or board-eligible and experienced ER doctors. As in any profession, skill levels do vary among doctors. Some are definitely better than others. Knowing a doctor's background and experience can't guarantee good medical care, but it certainly helps.

In many smaller hospitals and especially in more rural emergency rooms, residents in training are often used to cover the night and weekend hours and are known as moonlighters because they work these odd shifts. Basically, they work in the ER to make extra money. This is beneficial for smaller hospitals that need to provide around-the-clock doctor coverage for their emergency rooms, and it also helps the residents. The big problem is that many of these residents do not have the experience to handle many of the problems that may present to an ER. In fact, they may not even be primary care physicians, but specialists in obstetrics, orthopedics, pediatrics, or surgery. Of course some of the problems familiar to their specialty are often seen in the ER, but emergency medicine requires a broad base of knowledge that emphasizes the diagnosis, treatment, and care of acute medical problems in patients of many ages, different sexes, and from varying cultural backgrounds.

Let's give you an example. A woman comes to the ER complaining of chest pain. The ER doctor is a surgeon who is not trained in the subtle varying signs of heart attacks in women. He misdiagnoses the woman, and sends her home. Later that night, the woman has a massive heart attack and dies. Similarly, if an orthopedic resident is moonlighting and has to evaluate a pediatric patient with a high fever, she may miss the early signs of meningitis or pneumonia and fail to provide the proper treatment soon enough to prevent lifelong problems. These doctors may have the best of intentions, but it doesn't mean that they have the skill level needed to care for these problems adequately. Doctors know that when they, or their family members, go to an emergency room, they have to inquire about the training, background, and experience of the treating physician. You've got to know the background and training of those treating you.

Most physicians' ability to make the correct diagnosis is dependent upon their seeing or being exposed to patients who have had that same diagnosis in the past. If you haven't seen a particular medical problem previously, you may miss a particular diagnosis. The skill to make a diagnosis (especially a difficult one) often only comes with many years of experience and some mistakes (hopefully minor) that all doctors make in the course of dealing with patients. Because OB-GYN doctors don't see sick children and pediatricians don't see adults with chest pain, they will not be skilled in providing the best care for these problems, especially in more complex cases. It takes time to make a good physician. It also takes maturity to develop that intuition and insight that enables a doctor to make a difficult diagnosis when he is only given a few clues. It's almost impossible to make a correct diagnosis in a difficult case when it's outside his particular specialty area or field of expertise.

Be wary. Just because someone has *doctor* if front of her name does not automatically make her a good doctor or knowledgeable about areas of medicine outside of her expertise. As soon as you graduate from medical school, you can put M.D. after your name, but we personally would not want any first-year resident making a diagnosis on his or her own without consulting with a more experienced doctor. It takes experience to be the best doctor possible. We all learn from our mistakes and doctors are no different from other professionals. One of the good things about how doctors are trained is that they have others reviewing what they do. Unfortunately, this is often not the case when it comes to the delivery of care in rural ERs until it's too late.

Mark July 1 down in your mental calendar especially if you go to a teaching hospital. Why is this date so important? **July 1 is the date when the new residency-training year traditionally begins at teaching hospitals and when many new doctors just out of training are starting assignments at their new hospitals.** It's a time of considerable confusion and angst. Many nurses ask for time off during these first couple of weeks so that they don't have to deal with the new doctors who are so wet behind the ears. As a patient, you need to know that you just may be the first patient a new doctor has ever seen on his own after graduating from medical school. (This should be a very scary thought.) Fortunately, all teaching programs realize this and have set up mechanisms to supervise these beginning doctors.

Kevin's Comments

I can remember how scared I was when I began my residency. I had all this book knowledge from medical school but had no real experience in seeing and evaluating patients by myself. When I walked in to see that first patient on July 1, I was sure he could hear my heart racing and see my knees shaking. Somehow or other I got through it . . . and so did he. We both survived, as did all the patients I saw in the ER that first year. I've spoken to a number of doctors about their experiences with their first patients since then and they've all had that same scared feeling inside . . . no matter the apparent cool on the outside. Fortunately, we all had safety nets in the form of the older residents or our attending physicians who reviewed all of our cases and kept us from making any serious mistakes. Without that safety net, I, and other doctors, would have been terrified.

Here's our advice for you. Ask the doctor who is examining you how long she's been working in an ER and what is her particular specialty. If you feel uncomfortable asking the doctor about his or her credentials (as most of us would be), ask the nurse in the triage area or the nurse that brings you back to your examining room some basic information about the doctor who will be examining you or your family member. Here are some questions we'd suggest you ask:

- What is the background and training of the doctor who will be seeing me?

- Do you trust him/her?

- Would you go to see him/her if you were sick with a similar problem?

- Has he or she had much experience in evaluating a problem like mine?

In most cases, hospital staff will be very honest with you when faced with such questions. If you get evasive answers or are told not to worry about those sorts of things, you ought to be very cautious and should ask the doctor these questions yourself.

It's important for patients to get answers to these questions. It will either comfort you or make you more likely to ask more questions about what is being done for you and be insistent about getting additional testing or close follow-up when you leave the ER. If you're in a teaching hospital, insist on speaking to a more experienced attending physician personally before leaving the ER so that he hears your story directly. It's also an opportunity for you to ask questions that the younger doctor may not be able to answer in a way that helps you understand. ERs are hectic places and any doctor can miss things if feeling rushed or overworked. It never hurts to have an extra pair of eyes and another brain looking at your particular case. Doctors would do these things for their families . . . and you should too.

Does Your ER have Someone Experienced Reading X Rays, CT Scans, and MRIs on Nights or on Weekends?

Many of the problems that are seen in the ER require additional testing of various kinds to make a proper diagnosis. At larger hospitals—known as secondary or tertiary care hospitals—there is no problem having sufficient staff to provide laboratory and radiology department services round the clock. In many smaller hospitals, there are not enough patients to warrant the expense of having supporting personnel 24/7 for all the departments. What does this mean for you as a patient? Certain tests may not be done on a timely basis or may be delayed while support personnel are called to the hospital.

Picture a small hospital late at night. An auto accident victim with lots of trauma is brought to the ER. The emergency room doctor is concerned about abdominal trauma and wants to get a CT scan of the patient's abdomen to check for internal bleeding. He or she orders the CT scan but now has to wait until the technician gets out of bed, comes to the ER, and warms up the machine. Then either the ER doctor reads the CT (but maybe it's a pediatric resident who's moonlighting and has no clue about how to read the film) or the radiologist on call has to be called and brought into the hospital to read the film. All of this can mean a potentially deadly delay for the patient awaiting the results. If there is blood in the abdomen, a surgeon needs to be called immediately to evaluate the patient for possible exploratory surgery to find the source of internal bleeding. In any case, it's the patient who might suffer.

Some hospitals have the capability of sending images via telephone to radiologists in other institutions. This saves time and ensures that experienced physicians are reviewing the films. As a potential patient, explore the kind of coverage for radiology services your hospital has. What services does your hospital provide? If you don't know, then find out. You may just want to drive a bit farther to get better, faster care.

DON'T GO TO THE ER UNLESS IT'S AN EMERGENCY

Don't go to the ER if you can see your doctor for the same problem. Sounds simple enough, doesn't it? But for all the people who use the ER appropriately, there are a large number who abuse it. According to some studies, up to 50 percent of patients seen in an ER were nonemergencies and could easily have been treated in doctor's offices. It's these people who clog the system and help to create the long waits. You may wait for a while in your doctor's office, but it won't be as long as waiting in an emergency room, especially if you're there for a nonemergent medical problem. Generally, in a doctor's office, you will get more personal care and your doctor should know more about your past medical history, including the medicines you are taking. In the ER, this is often not the case.

 ## Christine's Comments

There are times, however, when it's best to go straight to the ER instead of your doctor's office.

A friend of mine called me the other day. She was visiting with her elderly aunt and during her visit, her aunt had taken ill. She described the symptoms to me over the phone and they sounded like classic symptoms of a stroke. I told her to call 911, get her aunt in an ambulance and get her to the hospital immediately. I told her that if her aunt was having a stroke, time was of the essence if the doctors were going to be able to give her as much help as possible.

What happened? The aunt's daughter came to get her mom and instead of taking her to the ER, took her to her family practitioner's office where they waited for about two hours . . . and then the family doctor told them to go to the emergency room. The doctors in the hospital told her that she had indeed

suffered a stroke. She survived it but clearly could have had a better outcome, had she been taken straight to the ER.

When you think you may be seriously ill, err to the side of caution and go straight to the ER. Do not be a hero. Do not be embarrassed to call 911. Paramedics and ambulances are designed to get you to the hospital ER quickly and safely. Do not worry what your neighbors and coworkers will think. Do not worry about how much money the ambulance will cost. Just get to the ER and let them save your life. Nothing else matters as much as that.

Obviously, all of us need to secure a primary care doctor . . . and not just any doctor. You need to make sure your doctor can find time for you in her busy schedule, especially on those occasions when you are really sick. You also should expect her to have someone taking after-hours call, or available when she will be out of town. Believe it or not, many doctors do not have these types of arrangements and simply dump patients on the ER when not in their offices. Initially, you may not speak to a doctor in their off-hours, but will often first speak to a nurse practitioner, physician's assistant, or a nurse. These medical personnel can handle most problems until the next day, when you can be seen in the office. (A recent study confirmed this fact.) If not, they can often arrange for some definitive care if your problem is more serious. This might include getting the doctor to call you directly or referring you to the ER. The bottom line: Get a doctor for yourself and for your family who is there when you need him.

HOW IMPORTANT IS IT TO GET TO THE ER QUICKLY IN CERTAIN CONDITIONS?

Two words: absolutely essential. The longer you wait to get to the ER in certain conditions, the greater the chances of something going seriously wrong or dying. Time can mean increasing trouble. Unfortunately, many people wait too long to get the emergency care they need. Most patients don't want to overreact, often wonder when it's appropriate to go to the ER, or when they should wait and simply monitor their condition.

Kevin's Comments

Frank S. was a fifty-five-year-old man whom I saw in the ER one morning around 7 A.M. During the middle of the night, he had begun to experience chest pain and difficulty breathing. He told me that it felt at first like an elephant was sitting on his chest. He was worried that it might be a heart attack, but because it was two in the morning, he didn't want to wake his wife, especially if it turned out to be a case of simple indigestion. It was bad enough that he waited, but then he did another stupid thing. He had his wife drive him to the ER. If you think you're having a heart attack, always call 911 and get taken by ambulance. Why? The paramedics can monitor your heart and treat dangerous, life-threatening arrhythmias (abnormal beats that keep your heart from pumping properly) as well as begin treatments that will help lessen the damage to your heart.

Unfortunately, it was a heart attack and Frank had some definite damage to his heart. He was put in the CCU, and it was touch and go for a while. If he had come into the ER when he first had his chest pain, we might have been able to save more of his heart muscle. As it was, he had so much damage to his heart that he went into heart failure while in the hospital.

I can't tell you how many times I've heard stories similar to this. Even after all these years and all the educational efforts to explain the importance of getting to the ER quickly when you think you might be having a heart attack, patients still wait, for the stupidest of reasons. I hate to say it, but men seem to be the worst when it comes to waiting or denying that something

serious is going on. (Women, don't start feeling good about yourselves, as I've seen many of you make the same kind of dumb mistakes.)

There are two important lessons that we all should learn from this case. First, get to an emergency room as soon as possible when you even think you might be having a heart attack. The sooner you begin treatment of a heart attack, the less likely you are to have damage to your heart, and the more likely you'll reduce the risk of dangerous complications like your chances for abnormal beats or heart failure. We know of too many cases in which people with heart attacks or strokes didn't make it to the ER in what's known as the "golden hour" of time, when the adverse-effects could have been reversed. As a result, they were left with a useless arm or leg or suffered severe heart damage.

Second, always call 911 and get the paramedics to bring you to the ER. They can begin evaluating and monitoring you as soon as possible. (They can also begin treatment if necessary.)

When to Go to the ER

There are certain signs and symptoms that should trigger an immediate trip to the ER. Some of these are:

Severe pain: Pain is always an indication that something is wrong. Pain can be unremitting like the chest pain of a heart attack or the rupture of an ectopic pregnancy. It can come in waves like the terrible pain associated with kidney stones. When there is the sudden onset of pain that does not go away quickly or pain that comes on slowly and persists, get to the ER.

High temperature: Fever (generally a temperature over 100 degrees Fahrenheit) is a good thing for the body and is actually a protective mechanism. Young children can tolerate much higher temperatures than adults. We've often seen temps of 104 to 106 degrees in children who are doing surprisingly well. Temperatures in that same range in adults would have them delirious. Fevers over 103 degrees that don't respond to antipyretics (temperature-reducing drugs) like acetaminophen (Tylenol and Datril) and ibuprofen (Advil and Motrin) should be evaluated in the ER.

Unconsciousness or change in mental status: When a person's mental condition becomes changed and they begin talking out of their heads and making no sense, or if they lose the ability to communicate, it is an extremely serious sign and the person should be seen by a doctor immediately. It can be caused by a number of things like head trauma, infection in the brain, or a stroke.

Chest pain or pressure in the chest: Many people wait way too long before coming to the ER when they have a heart attack. Persistent chest pain, pressure in the chest, or back and chest pain at the same time should have you calling the ambulance and getting someone directly to the ER. Delay can be deadly.

Slurred speech, drooping on one side of the face, or loss of the use of a limb: These are all signs of a stroke and should immediately send someone to the ER.

Severe persistent headache different from others: Many people get headaches and they are almost never a serious problem. But some headaches may signal the onset of a stroke or a hemorrhage in the brain, especially when they are abrupt in onset and are worse than any other headache you might have had in the past.

Uncontrolled or unexplained bleeding: Nosebleeds are a good example of the former problem while vomiting up blood (GI or gastrointestinal bleeding) is an example of the latter condition. Most bleeding can be stopped with direct pressure in ten to fifteen minutes. If bleeding doesn't stop in that time period, then seek help in your local ER.

Clearly, in the case of medical problems like a heart attack and stroke, treating them sooner rather than later can make all the difference when it comes to a cure or prevention of long-term consequences.

Strokes and Golden Hour of Time for Treatment

In patients with stroke symptoms, there is a "golden hour" (actually three hours) when the appropriate medicines must be given to improve the chances of reversing the blockage of a particular kind of stroke called an ischemic stroke. Ischemic strokes (blockage to an artery in the brain) account for 80 percent of strokes, while hemorrhagic strokes (a blood vessel bursts and bleeds into the brain) account for the remaining 20 percent. The data clearly indicates that failure to get the thrombolytic agent (one that breaks up the blood clot) TPA into a patient's system within three hours decreases the chances of reversing the symptoms of the stroke. If a patient has lost the use of their arm and leg on one side because of a stroke, getting rapid treatment increases the odds of reversing this problem . . . but only when treated in those first few hours. New data also shows that getting to the ER and receiving the thrombolytic medicine within ninety minutes greatly reduces the chances of side effects from the clot-busting medicine.

The American Stroke Association fully understands the importance of being treated promptly and so is trying to help educate patients about the need for the utmost speed in beginning treatment when a stroke occurs. They advocate the three R's—Reduce, Recognize, and Respond.

Reduce asks that patients look at the risk factors that contribute to stroke and then actively work to eliminate or minimize them. This means getting blood pressure under control, getting rid of tobacco, and paying attention to diabetes.

Recognize the signs and symptoms of a stroke in yourself and others. A recent survey of U.S. adults revealed that 97 percent of those questioned could not identify a single symptom of stroke. If you don't recognize it, then you'll never be able to react quickly enough.

Respond by taking action. The only action that should be taken is to go to the nearest emergency room that can provide the medicines that will help reduce the long-term effects of stroke.

CHILDREN AND THE ER . . . THEY'RE NOT JUST LITTLE ADULTS

Imagine this: Your four-year-old child has been vomiting and running a fever for twenty-four hours. It's 1 A.M. and she's beginning to look extremely sick, so you're now very worried. You can't reach your family doctor, so you decide to take your child to the emergency room. You've never had to go to the ER before, but you live in a large city with three hospitals. Each has an ER, so you assume that it doesn't make a difference which one you go to. How different could the care your child will get at each be?

Stop and pay very close attention. The care you and your family receive in hospital emergency rooms can be vastly different . . . and even potentially life-threatening, especially for your children.

In 1993, the Institute of Medicine in Washington, D.C., the same group that wrote the 1999 report warning of ninety thousand unnecessary deaths in hospitals (see Chapter 4), issued Emergency Medical Services for Children. This four-hundred-plus-page report clearly detailed the need for major fixes in the current system of EMS and emergency room care if children and adults were treated properly and safely. Many of the problem areas that were detailed in the report ten years ago remain problems today in many hospitals. People cannot assume that hospital ERs are equal in the type of and level of care that they deliver. It just isn't true and patients need to very conscious of this as they seek emergency care.

As you've read earlier, emergency rooms can be dangerous places, but especially so if you are a child. Why? One of the biggest reasons is that many physicians who work in the ER are not trained to treat children. The margin of error when you make a mistake is smaller in children. Some emergency rooms treat so few children who are really sick that they don't have the proper equipment for caring for them and the dosages of medicines may not be as familiar to doctors or nurses.

Dr. Joel Cohen, an ER doctor in Mesa, Arizona, has written an excellent book entitled *ER: Enter at Your Own Risk*. He clearly states that some hospitals are much better than others in treating pediatric emergencies. Dr. Cohen and Dr. Stanley Inkelis, the director of the American Academy of Pediatrics (AAP) subcommittee on pediatric emergency care in nonchildren's hospitals, developed some questions for helping you evaluate your hospital's preparedness in this area. You can also go to *www.ems-c.org* to download *Child and Adolescent Health Care Services: A Community Assessment Guide* to help you better evaluate the state of your hospital's pediatric care.

Here are some of the questions that you should ask your ER.

What kinds of doctors treat children in the ER?

As we discussed earlier in the chapter, many ERs are not staffed with physicians trained or skilled in emergency medicine, much less pediatric emergency medicine. Ideally, if you have a sick child or a child with an emergent condition, you want them cared for by a doctor or physician extender trained in pediatric emergencies. Think about it. If you had a serious gynecologic problem, wouldn't you want to be cared for by a specialty-trained gynecologist? If you had a bad fracture of a bone or a severe joint injury, wouldn't you want an orthopedist handling the problem? If that's the case, why don't we demand the same kind of specialty care for our children in emergencies?

If in the evenings or on weekends, your hospital is staffed by moonlighting doctors not necessarily skilled in emergency medicine and you know of another hospital that has emergency room specialists, which would you prefer? It doesn't take a rocket scientist to get the correct answer. How many surgeons treat lots of children? How many OB-GYN, internists, or orthopedic doctors see many children? The answer is clearly not many, yet these are some of the specialists that sometimes staff emergency rooms. They are rarely as adept at diagnosing and understanding children's medical problems, as are family doctors, ER specialists, or pediatricians.

Using "moonlighters" to staff emergency rooms is very common and you need to determine what the staffing practice is at your particular hospital and at surrounding hospitals. Some moonlighting doctors can be extremely adept at caring for children so find out what their specialties are. Sometimes you may not have a choice, but when you do, take the specialist with the most experience in treating children's problems. It probably makes little difference with minor problems, but it can mean the difference between life and death in more serious problems.

Please pay very close attention here. Find out from the ER staff at your hospital what experience the ER doctor-on-duty has in treating children. If not much, be very careful or ask for a second opinion from another doctor.

Does the ER have the necessary pediatric equipment?

If you were asked to cook a meal without the right kinds of pots or pans, how comfortable would you be? If you were asked to repair a leaky faucet or running toilet without the proper tools, it would be, at the very least, extremely difficult. Working on modern-day cars is virtually impossible without some very sophisticated equipment. People, especially children, are

Kevin's comments

About twenty-five years ago, I was moonlighting in a small ER in rural North Carolina when a child was brought in late at night with severe respiratory problems. The child needed to be intubated (have a small tube put down her throat to help her breathe), but when the nurse opened the emergency cart to find the piece of equipment I needed (an endotracheal tube), there were no pediatric sizes. We had to get the night nurse to rush down to central supply. It was a horrible moment and had me feeling panicked. Fortunately, the right size was found and the child survived. In most cases with children, you can't use adult-size equipment. It just doesn't work. A hospital needs to have the proper pediatric equipment as well as the staff skilled in using it.

no different. Having the right tools and equipment is essential to taking the best care of children.

You can't get a correct blood pressure reading in very large or obese adults without an oversize blood pressure cuff. You also can't get a true blood pressure in children unless you use a pediatric-size cuff. If you find yourself in either of these situations, ask that the staff get a correct cuff for your situation. A wrong blood pressure reading can significantly alter your treatment, to the point of getting medicines you don't need. Don't let this happen to your child.

Another good example of the need for the right equipment for children is the use of neck braces in trauma cases. In those rare instances in which you might have to immobilize a child with potential neck problems, a cervical collar is used to prevent further injury to the neck and possibly avoid paralysis. A survey of one hundred emergency departments in 1998 and 1999 revealed that only 43 percent of respondents had these needed collars in the ER. The bottom line: Children are not little adults and cannot use adult equipment. It could mean the difference between life and death in certain instances.

The American Academy of Pediatrics has a Web site, *www.aap.org*, that provides a list of the kind of equipment that an ER that sees children should have on hand. Get this list and then call or go by the local ER and determine whether or not they have it.

Does the ER have a separate treatment area for children?

Can you imagine a young child sitting in the ER waiting to be treated for an earache and in comes a person with a gunshot wound, or a large laceration with blood all over their clothes, or maybe a loudmouthed drunk who's cursing and belligerent to those caring for him? It's bad enough for other adults to see some of the things that walk or are carried through the emergency room doors, but just imagine what it would be like for children.

Most children's hospitals have separate treatment areas for children in their emergency departments, but many community hospitals don't have the space or haven't given this much thought. One immediate advantage of having a separate area is that all the necessary children's equipment can be kept in one place.

Who does triage in the ER for children?

When you come to the ER, there is a person assigned to triage patients and determine their level of need. The sickest patients are seen first, those less acute next, and finally, those with nonacute problems. In most hospitals, this job is assigned to nurses, since they should have some skill at determining who is more ill. The problem in some hospitals is that less skilled nurses are often given this task, and in some cases, technicians.

Here's the problem. Unless you are trained specifically in evaluating sick children, you can often miss the severity of their illness, especially if they are sleeping or crying. Children can't talk to you like adults can, so it's important that the person doing the triage be skilled. If you go to the ER, ask the person admitting you and your child what their background is and how comfortable they feel evaluating children. If they aren't well skilled, ask that someone else check out your child if they are very ill and are not taken back to see the doctor soon.

Another group that is often underevaluated by those performing triage as well as the doctors caring for them are persons from other countries who speak English poorly or not at all. Communications between doctors and patients can be bad enough when both parties speak English. Throw in a foreign language and you've added additional opportunities for miscommunication. Many hospitals now provide translators in emergency room situations. They can be staff members or the hospital has an arrangement with outside agencies. If you need services such as these, ask that the hospital find a translator even if over the phone. After all, it's your health that's on the line.

---

10 RULES DOCTOR KNOW ABOUT
The ER . . . And You Should Too

---

1. **Don't downplay your symptoms:** The worst thing that you can do with your ER doctor is to minimize your symptoms because it lulls the doctor into not taking your complaints as seriously. As a result,

your doctor may do less aggressive testing than is required. Here's a good example: If you have abdominal pain and downplay it, the doctor may not perform a CT scan that could help to diagnose your condition. If you make light of your chest pain, the doctor may be less likely to admit you to the hospital for observation when it just might be what's needed to save your life. Downplaying your symptoms is just like lying. It does no one any good. It's especially true when you're in an emergency situation.

Kevin's Comments

One day in the ER, a healthy-appearing, muscular man of forty-one years came in complaining of chest pain on occasion. He looked fit, like a bodybuilder. He mentioned that he was in the ER because his wife wanted his chest pain checked out. He didn't appear worried about it and denied any of the usual symptoms associated with cardiac pain. I ordered an electrocardiogram (ECG) and went to speak to his wife.

I always try to speak to family. The patient's wife told me that his pain was so bad at times that it almost doubled him over and that he'd put a fist to his chest when it happened (a sign often associated with heart pain). She also told me that his father had died of a heart attack in his early forties and his older brother had had a heart attack in his forties as well.

I went back to see my patient and his ECG showed only minor changes. Because of his history, I contacted the internal medicine doctor on call. He agreed to admit my patient and perform a cardiac stress test on the treadmill the next day. My patient couldn't go for more than a few minutes before he had chest pain and marked changes on his cardiogram. They did an emergency heart catheterization that same day and he had severe blockages in three arteries leading to his heart. The next day (the second day after I saw him in the ER) he had four-vessel heart bypass surgery. The man would likely have suffered a serious heart attack if he hadn't come to the ER.

My patient had minimized his symptoms and this could have cost him his life if I hadn't taken the time to talk to his family. Patients often don't tell us the full story because they're trying to be tough or are in denial. You're not helping anyone when you do this.

2. **Bring family members or friends with you to the ER:** No, it's not for social reasons. The key reason for bringing someone with you to the ER (ideally it should be someone who knows you) is that when you're sick, you often can't remember what's said or you may leave out important parts of your medical history. Family and friends can help to keep you honest. Another reason for bringing someone with you: If you receive certain medication while in the ER, you shouldn't be driving. Family members can also remind you of instructions for medicines as well as when and how to get your follow-up care.

3. **If you have a personal physician, call her and tell her that you are going to the ER. Don't wait for her to return your call before heading for the ER as a time delay can make a difference in the outcome:** By calling your personal doctor, she is alerted to the fact that you have a serious medical problem. She can often speed your way to the front of the line and may have some orders waiting for you when you arrive. It's nice if you get a quick call back, but if your doctor is busy, don't wait if you have some of the symptoms that we've outlined previously.

4. **Bring a list of all your medicines with you, including dosages:** Try to remember "Grab and Go." Grab your bottles of medicine and go to the ER. There is nothing worse (or more dangerous) for a doctor than caring for someone and not having any idea of what medicines they are taking. It's too easy to have drug interactions that can cause serious health problems if a wrong medicine is prescribed. The

majority of patients seen in the ER have no idea what they're taking. Make a list or bring the bottles with you. Don't leave it to chance because it can kill you.

5. **Get written instructions. Read them and make sure you understand them:** Never leave the ER without written instructions. When you do get them, make sure you understand them all. If not, ask for clarification, and don't leave until you get it. Aftercare can sometimes be just as important as the initial care. Oftentimes, a patient will present an initial set of symptoms that will lead the doctor toward one diagnosis, but within twelve to twenty-four hours, the symptoms change significantly and another diagnosis turns out to be the correct one. Another reason for seeing another doctor is to make sure you're not worsening or having some problems as a result of the initial care. If you have a cast put on for a broken bone, there can be problems with swelling that can cause further problems like nerve damage. This is why follow-up care is critical. Your ER doctor should provide very specific care on how to treat your injury, what to look for that might indicate that your condition is worsening, and what to do if it does worsen.

6. **Ask questions so that you understand all aspects of your care:** Doctors know that the only dumb question is the one not asked. If you don't understand something, ask the doctor. If the doctor doesn't explain so that you understand, then ask the nurse to clarify. If the doctor doesn't answer your questions, tell the manager of the ER. If that doesn't work, ask for the hospital administrator on call.

7. **Make sure that you get a doctor to follow up with if you are no better:** Many times the emergency room is only the first step in your care. If you have a broken bone, you will need casting and close supervision by an orthopedic specialist until the bone heals. If you have abdominal pain, you may not require surgery initially, but in twenty-four to forty-eight hours, if things worsen or get no better,

you might. If you don't have a doctor of your own to follow your care, don't leave without the name of a physician and how to contact them.

8. **Ask about your medicines and get your prescriptions filled immediately:** How well do you think a medicine can work if you don't get it into your body? You're right, not at all. But let us assure you that we've seen too many patients who leave the ER with prescriptions and never get them filled (or maybe they wait a day or two). They then call the ER all upset because they're not getting any better. They then have the nerve to ask for a new prescription for something else. Sorry, folks, but that dog just isn't going to hunt with us. You have to take your medicine exactly as prescribed or you're not helping yourself. Make sure you understand what you are to do before you leave the ER, how you should expect to feel if you're getting better, and how long it should take. Remember . . . you didn't get sick in a day and you won't get better in a day.

9. **Do your homework about the doctor you're referred to. He may be the doctor on call but may not be the best doctor for you:** Hospitals have to have backup physicians on call. They don't have to be the best physicians. They just have to be available because they are on the hospital staff. You might get lucky and be referred to one of the better members of the hospital staff in the specialty you require, but you never know. What should you do? You need to make the same inquiries that you would if selecting a physician for the first time (look at our instructions in Chapter 1). Make a decision about follow-up only after checking out the doctor you are referred to. If you don't have time to check out the new doctor adequately, then get to that first appointment because follow-up is so important. After all, one appointment does not have to mean a long-term commitment. The important thing is just to get to a doctor for care. And who knows, you may just really like this new doctor.

10. **Don't wait to follow up if you're no better or your symptoms worsen:** Despite the best efforts of the ER doctor, your child remains sick and may be worsening after twenty-four hours. You're not sure what to do. Let us tell you. Follow up with your regular doctor or with some other doctor as soon as possible. You don't need to wait, even if the ER doctor said to seek help in two to three days. Here's a great example of this. Patients with appendicitis will often present a first symptom of stomach pain or pain around their liver. If the ER doctor sees you with this early sign, he may miss the appendicitis and make some other diagnosis. In twelve to twenty-four hours, this pain can move to the right lower side and clearly signal appendicitis even to a first-year medical student. You know your situation better than anyone. Pay attention to your signs and symptoms. If you're worsening or have some serious medical symptoms as we outlined above, don't wait. Get back to the ER or to another doctor as soon as possible.

Summary

Doctors know where the best ER is and which ones have the most skilled physicians. You need the best doctors in emergency situations. The time to check out where to go for you and your family is now . . . before any emergency. Asking some key questions during your visit to the ER could mean the difference between living and dying. Follow the instructions you receive in the ER to the letter and don't be afraid to return if your condition is worsening.

CHAPTER EIGHT

CARDIOVASCULAR DISEASE: THE BIGGEST KILLER IN THE UNITED STATES

Heart disease is truly a nondiscriminating killer. It is the number one cause of death in the United States among whites, blacks, men, and women. Despite our knowledge of this disease, death rates remain close to 50 percent and are double that of cancer, the next leading cause of death.

Do you ever wonder why some people with normal cholesterol and no other apparent risk factors for heart disease suddenly drop dead of a heart attack? Are you aware that a great deal of the whole theory behind what leads to heart attacks is being turned upside down right at this very moment? How come certain doctors are advising some of their patients to take a combination of vitamins to reduce high levels of an element that can damage your arteries and lead to heart attacks? What's the latest information about the "new biology" of heart disease? What are the commonly known risk factors for cardiovascular disease that *you can control?* After all, there are some risks that you can control, and others that you can't. We'll make sure you know the difference.

We don't plan on recounting many of the facts and risks that you already know, but will emphasize what's new and different. Some doctors are aware of a whole new way of preventing and treating heart disease, but most have no idea about these latest major breakthroughs. We think that some of what we tell you in this chapter will shock and surprise you. Your physicians or other health care professionals may make light of what we are telling you, or say that there's not enough evidence to justify changes in how you are treated. We don't believe this . . . and neither do many prominent physicians who are making changes and caring for patients in new ways.

We hope that what you learn here will reduce your risk of heart disease and may save your life. We hope you'll take what you read here to your doctor, because if he is not following these guidelines, or is not telling you about these latest advances in the treatment of heart disease and blood pressure problems, then you're not getting the best possible medical care. This one chapter alone can do more than anything else you'll read to reduce your chances of dying from the number one killer in the United States. We hope you'll take this information to heart.

WOMEN NOT GETTING THE CARE THEY NEED: IS MEDICINE FAILING WOMEN?

Christina was a forty-one-year-old woman of Mediterranean descent who visited her gynecologist every year or two for her routine health checkups. On this particular occasion, her gynecologist had told her that he wanted to do a complete workup. As a result, she had a Pap smear, an ultrasound to check for ovarian cancer, a mammogram to check for breast cancer, and an endometrial biopsy to screen for uterine cancer. All of her tests came back normal, so Christina was tremendously relieved and declared herself in great health to all of our friends. She felt she had done all she could to ensure the maintenance of her health.

> **Heart disease is the number one killer in the U.S. It kills more women and men than all other causes of death put together.**

Isn't this a wonderful story and one that many women patients could relate to? The answers to these questions are a surprising *no* and *yes*. Many women can identify with this scenario because all the medical care that the majority of women in the United States get is from their gynecologists. But shouldn't it be reassuring that the patient's doctor in this scenario did all the right tests for cancer . . . and more than many doctors might do?

Think again. This is wonderful care if all that you're concerned about is cancer, but that's not what's killing most women.

Heart disease is the number one killer in the United States. It kills more women and men than all other causes of death put together. Heart disease is the number one killer and strokes are the number three killer, and both of these diseases are included as a part of cardiovascular disease. This data has been true for years, but surprisingly, in a survey conducted by the American Heart Association in 2000, 62 percent of the female respondents identified cancer as their chief health threat. Only 8 percent knew heart disease kills more women—about two times as many as all cancers combined. Hello, it's time to wake up and learn more about the risk factors for cardiovascular disease and stroke. These are the diseases that are going to kill more of you than anything else will.

Let's just be blunt about it:

Relying only on your gynecologist for your medical care may be killing you. Believe it or not, a woman's OB-GYN doctor may be contributing to the underdetection and improper treatment of heart disease. How? Many women use their OB-GYN doctor as their primary care physician. An OB-GYN is fine for many things, but in the time allotted for a routine ob-gyn examination they do not have the time and in many cases, the specialized training, to detect or care for heart disease. This can often lead to late diagnoses, missed diagnoses, or failure to provide good preventive care. It's not a failing on the part of the gynecologist because they're specialists in diseases affecting the female reproductive organs—not in cardiovascular disease. And even if an OB-GYN is board certified to be a primary care physician, many women are not getting all the essential medical tests needed at an annual exam (see Chapter 3).

Why can't women just demand more heart tests from their gynecologists? There's a basic problem with this. Gynecologists aren't trained in the subtleties of cardiovascular tests and the proper response to abnormal tests, so women would often be shortchanged even if they had more testing. Would the average gynecologist know how to identify the early signs of heart disease or how to interpret the various tests used to screen for it, and then be able to prescribe the required medicines or care? Maybe, given enough time, but with busy practices and managed care necessitating less time spent with each patient, OB-GYNs barely have enough time to perform a thorough gynecological exam, no less cover anything else. Besides, just because an OB-GYN learned about heart disease in medical school, doesn't mean he is the best person to care for your heart. After all, orthopedic surgeons learned how to do PAP smears in medical school, but you wouldn't go to them for your annual gynecological exam, would you?

What do doctors know to do and we think you should do? Think of care below your waist for gynecologists and think of your family doctor or internist for the care of the rest of you. We realize that this might be a bit of an oversimplification, but we hope it makes the point with you. Women can keep going to their gynecologists, but they also need to begin seeing a primary care doctor skilled in the prevention and treatment of cardiovascular disease.

Heart Disease and Women

Here's something that's going to surprise you and may not make many women very happy. Until recently, research into heart disease and its treatment has used men in almost all the clinical trials. Researchers took the results of the studies on men and simply extrapolated the findings to women. It seems ludicrous now, but that's what was done for years. As a result, heart disease in women is largely misunderstood by both laypeople and many health care providers. But it's now clear that there are big differences between the sexes when it comes to the onset of symptoms, the diagnosis, and the treatment of heart disease.

One of the big differences may be in the levels of circulating estrogen that women have until they go through menopause. As long as women have good levels of estrogen in their system, the risk of heart disease is rare in comparison to men of similar ages. But when women begin to go through menopause and estrogen levels begin to fall (often in the late forties and early fifties), their arteries begin to change and the risk of cardiovascular disease becomes more like a man's. The rate of heart attacks begins to increase as estrogen decreases, and by around age sixties, the risk for women becomes equal to men.

Most women simply do not believe that they are at risk for heart disease. They think it is someone else's problem. The women most in denial are younger women. The truth is that more and more younger women are developing early signs of heart disease. Higher levels of smoking and obesity in younger women are partially to blame, along with a significant increase in women with diabetes. Diabetes alone increases the risk of heart disease by two to five times. Some risk factors affect women more severely than men. In fact, smoking and diabetes seem to totally counteract whatever protective benefits that being a younger woman with high levels of naturally circulating estrogen brings. Women may also be more adversely affected by stress, which they feel differently than men do, and it may be a contributing factor to the increased incidence of heart problems.

Another major problem for women is that they often have different symptoms of heart disease than men do. Men get the classic signs of chest pain often radiating to the jaw or down the left arm, shortness of breath, cold sweats, and nausea. Women, on the other hand, may get back pain, unexplained fatigue, shortness of breath not associated with pain and abdominal pain. Another big difference between men and women is that in this one instance, men may be more aware of their symptoms and seek treatment. Why? Men are constantly on alert and think that they might be suffering a heart attack, even when they feel perfectly fine, probably because they know lots of friends or coworkers who have had the experience. Women rarely have friends who have had a heart attack, especially prior to the age of forty-five.

Women need to be more suspicious of changes in their health, especially as they get older. But even younger women need to be vigilant. Last year, Oprah devoted a whole show to stories of younger women who had symptoms of a heart attack that were initially ignored by themselves and by their doctors. Heart disease is not something that women think about right away especially if the symptoms are unusual and they are of a younger age . . . but they should.

The problem is made worse by the fact that until recently, many doctors weren't trained to recognize these different, subtle signs and symptoms in women. Even today, many doctors are unaware of these subtle symptoms of heart disease in women. As a result, women often get fewer tests for heart disease than men do. It's not surprising that when women feel the signs of a heart attack and finally get to the hospital, it takes a lot longer for doctors and nurses to diagnose their problem. Sometimes, this delay can be deadly, because it can make women too sick to qualify for certain lifesaving treatments, like the clot-buster medications that have the ability to stop a heart attack in its tracks. What should women do if they go to the ER or to their doctors and they are concerned about heart disease? They must talk to their doctors and insist that they get whatever tests are necessary to check it.

The Problem of Heart Disease Detection in Women

Detecting heart disease is very different for men and women. Often, as in our make-believe scenario, gynecologists will prescribe mammography and Pap smears, but will fail to order stress tests, electrocardiograms, or blood tests. Very simply, prevention varies by sex (the popular name for this in medicine is gender-specific medicine).

Some tests are simply not as effective for women as they are for men. To illustrate our point, let's use a popular example. Treadmill tests are considered the gold standard or best noninvasive test for the detection of heart disease, but it is just not useful for many women. The data indicate that treadmill tests are 90 percent accurate in men but only 42 percent accurate in women. Women often exercise less than men, so they can't get to the maximal level of functioning on the treadmill to generate a meaningful test.

Another problem is that the cause of heart attack in men and women can be very different, and the test used to detect impending heart attack in men is useless for many women. In men, cholesterol plaques account for 90 percent of the blockages to the coronary arteries of the heart. The problem in men is easy to detect by the "ultimate" test for heart disease—the cardiac catheterization. When the cardiac catheter is put into the arteries of the heart and dye is injected, the blockages in men are easily seen. However, true blockage accounts for only one-third of heart attacks in women. When women develop a blockage to one of the coronary arteries of the heart and have a heart attack, it's often caused by a spasm of the coronary artery. When the artery goes into spasm, the heart doesn't get enough blood flow, and then bingo, you have a heart attack. (One major triggering factor for this vasospasm is eating a meal heavy in fat. This spasm can occur four to six hours after the meal.) The vasospasm that causes the problem in women is often very difficult to detect even with a cardiac catheterization. Their coronary arteries are very often clean, without the visible evidence of any narrowing.

One indication that more women may be allowing their heart disease go undetected is the number of women having heart surgery and angioplasty compared to the number of men. For instance, in 1998, more than twice as many men had bypass surgery than women (396,000 vs. 158,000). It's also true for angioplasties . . . twice as many men have these procedures as have women.

The good news? New studies are finding that women who avail themselves of the latest advances in balloon angioplasty to open up dangerously narrowed arteries usually have successful results. This is partly because these tests are now being designed for women. In the past, catheters and stents were all made in the "one size fits all" model. No surprise, they were designed by men to fit men's larger arteries. Because of that, women suffered far more complications and a much higher risk of death from angioplasties. Also, amazingly until a few years ago, doctors used to prescribe the same doses of the blood thinner heparin for men and women, leading to greater internal bleeding in women.

Trust us, it's not that women don't have heart disease; it is just going undetected or they are not getting the same treatment.

WHAT DOCTORS KNOW ABOUT
Heart Disease . . . And You Should Too

---

1. Coronary artery disease (CAD) and strokes account for almost 65 percent of all deaths in both men and women.

2. Many of the risk factors for CAD and stroke are the same and are controllable with good medical care.

3. Millions of people are not receiving the proper treatment for reducing the risk factors associated with heart disease.

4. Women need to see a doctor who can evaluate and treat heart disorders.

5. Persons with a family history of early heart attack or stroke should pay particular attention to controlling their other risk factors.

6. Seventy percent of all deaths from heart disease are lifestyle related, so the choices you make in your life can have a real impact on your particular risk.

7. The new biology of heart disease indicates that inflammation is as important a risk factor for cardiovascular disease as is cholesterol.

THE NEW BIOLOGY OF HEART ATTACKS: INFLAMMATION AND HEART ATTACKS

Approximately 50 percent of heart attacks and strokes occur in people without any obvious risk factors like high blood pressure or high cholesterol. Patients were walking out of the doctor's office with a clean bill of health and would later have a massive heart attack. Doctor's knew they had to be missing something.

Until recently, it was thought that most heart attacks occurred when a complete blockage of a coronary artery (the arteries supplying blood to the heart) prevented blood from getting to a portion of the heart. The bigger the area of the heart not receiving blood flow, the more damage to the heart, and the greater risk of the patient dying. When researchers examined the plaques causing the blockages in people's arteries, they found that they were made up primarily of cholesterol. That's why most heart disease treatments have focused on reducing cholesterol in the plaques, or in more severe cases, bypassing these plaques with surgery.

But times they are a-changing, and new research has uncovered some radical findings. Dr. Peter Libby of the Harvard Medical School suggests that there is a "new biology" for heart attacks that sees inflammation within the vessel wall as potentially a greater contributing cause to heart attacks than cholesterol blockages. Libby believes that "the new biology leads to a new therapeutic goal to stabilize lesions rather than to extirpate, bypass, squash or stent them."

Let us translate what he's trying to say in plain English because it's extremely important. We no longer should focus our efforts on bypass surgery, angioplasties, or reducing the size of cholesterol plaques, but rather should work to help keep cholesterol plaques from breaking apart and triggering the inflammation that triggers a big clot in the artery leading to the heart. Whoa! Now that's a radical departure from how most physicians' approach coronary heart disease. Currently, we use angioplasties and coronary bypass surgeries to try to prevent or reduce the risk of heart disease when the future could require even simpler therapies to accomplish the same goal. The bottom line: High levels of inflammation in the body (as judged by high levels of the high-sensitivity C-reactive protein blood test, HSCRP) will now be considered one of the major risk factors for heart attacks and strokes in the new biology of cardiovascular disease.

According to the new biology theory, the degree of blockage (*stenosis* is the medical term for this) in the coronary arteries is *not* the key factor in cardiovascular disease; what is essential is stabilizing the plaques that exist around the arteries in the heart and controlling the amount of inflammation in a person's body. One of the biggest problems with heart disease is that it's not always seen on cardiac catheterization (sticking dye into the arteries of the heart) or when a person has a stress test because blockage inside the artery isn't always the problem. About 60 percent of men and 45 percent of women had no symptoms prior to sudden death or their first heart attack; plaque was present but hadn't caused a narrowing of the artery. When a plaque ruptures, a whole cascade of events occurs, and this causes heart attack. This is why this new biology of heart disease is so important. We need to keep cholesterol plaques stable and prevent them rupturing. Physicians will need to learn a new way to detect disease and treat it. You need to find the doctors that understand this new biology.

Let's look at what inflammation is and what causes it. Inflammation is a part of our bodies' natural defense system and occurs in response to an injury or to a chemical exposure. Injury can be caused by smoking or in response to some bacteria invading our system when we get an infection.

Diabetes and obesity also produce proteins that stimulate the inflammatory response in our bodies.

In recent studies, periodontal or gum disease has also been found to cause high levels of inflammation and increase a person's risk of heart disease almost two to three times above those without gum disease. Even when cholesterol levels were normal, persons with untreated periodontal disease had twice the risk of heart disease than did those without this problem. It appears that the same bacteria causing the gum disease can travel silently, like a stealth bomber, and invade your arterial walls, setting up a chronic inflammation. If this goes untreated, the results can be deadly.

C-Reactive Protein (CRP), Inflammation, and Your Risk of Heart Disease

The next logical question, and the one you're probably asking yourself now is: "How do I know if I have high levels of inflammation in my body? Unfortunately, you might not know you have it. You can have no symptoms, feel perfectly well, and appear the picture of health. This means you can be at risk for a sudden heart attack or stroke and not even know it.

Fortunately, there is a simple blood test costing about $20 that can tell if you have problems with inflammation. This test measures levels of C-reactive protein (CRP) in your blood. CRP is a protein that our liver makes in response to chronic irritations or injury. The level of CRP gives us a total cumulative measurement of systemic inflammation that can be caused by a wide range of injurious stressors. It isn't a specific inflammatory marker for injury to the heart but it is a general marker of a patient's overall state of inflammation much like a thermometer measures body temperature. There is now a newer version of this test called the high-sensitivity C-reactive protein (HSCRP) that is more specific than CRP. These tests are going to be particularly valuable for younger (pre-middle age) adults who don't have big red flags waving obvious risk factors to their physician.

Now you're probably saying, "So, what's the big deal about this CRP?"

Well, there's a really big deal about CRP and it's about to get a lot bigger. Women with high levels of CRP have a four times higher rate of heart disease than do women with normal levels of the blood test. Men with elevated levels of CRP have twice the risk of heart attacks and three times the risk of stroke than do men with normal levels of it. Here's the most important part of all this. People with normal levels of cholesterol and elevated levels of inflammation measured by CRP levels had twice the risk of heart attacks than those with normal levels of CRP. Cholesterol may be part of the problem for some people, but it's certainly not a major one for others.

There's some good news/bad news with the new biology of inflammation. The bad news is we get no warning signs or symptoms when our HSCRP is elevated. The good news is we can test for it and then take action if our HSCRP is elevated. By working with your doctor, you can begin to attack the specific problem causing your body's inflammatory reaction to gear up. It might be diabetes or high levels of cholesterol or periodontal disease. You have to eliminate the root cause of the inflammation to reduce your risk.

Treatment and Future Research

Obviously, the first line of treatment is to eliminate obvious risks. Diet and exercise can lower CRP dramatically. If you control your diabetes, the inflammatory reaction will be reduced markedly. Aspirin can also reduce CRP levels. Common cholesterol-lowering drugs also seems to be effective. In clinical trials in which specific cholesterol-lowering drugs known as the statins (e.g., Lipitor, Prevecol, Mevacor) were used, the blockage in patients' arteries was reduced only slightly, but despite this, the risk of heart attacks was decreased by 70 percent or more. Because the statin drugs also decrease inflammation, it is believed that reducing the amount of inflammation in the arteries may have been responsible for a remarkable drop in the number of heart attacks.

Other data lead scientists to believe that by treating patients with long-acting antibiotics, they can reduce the development of plaque buildup and rupture within arteries. A very recent study showed that the antibiotic doxycycline could reduce CRP levels by 50 percent. Although earlier we warned about the overuse of antibiotics, in this case the benefits may strongly outweigh the risks. However, you have to use narrow-spectrum antibiotics and these should not be used as a primary treatment, but only after many other things have been tried. The long-term use of antibiotics is certainly not advised for everyone, and it is not a commonly accepted practice, but we predict it's one we're likely to see more of in the future. Research is also under way to evaluate whether or not persons treated with anti-inflammatory drugs long-term may be at reduced risk.

C-Reactive Protein: FAQs

After getting my C-reactive protein levels tested, do I still need to pay attention to the traditional risk factors for heart disease?

You'd better believe it. These new findings should not affect the way we should be dealing with the traditional risk factors for cardiovascular disease. We still need to keep blood pressure within normal and healthy ranges, keep diabetes controlled, keep our cholesterol under control and keep our weight down.

What this new information tells us is that inflammation should be considered another risk factor that needs to be controlled like any other. Controlling inflammation is similar to high blood pressure and elevated cholesterol in that we usually have no symptoms associated with it to warn us when we're in trouble. With inflammation, we'll only discover we are at risk with a blood test called C-reactive protein which measures our total body burden of inflammation.

How important is it to measure the inflammation in my body using this new blood test?

Because the type of inflammation measured by the high sensitivity C-reactive protein blood test produces no symptoms in people, it is important to be tested to know what your risk may be.

What can I do to reduce elevated levels of inflammation in my body if I have them?

Inflammation is deadly and it needs to be controlled no matter the risk factor. You need to work with your physician and your dentist—together—to find out the source of your inflammation. Only then can you find the best treatment for you. Being obese can produce high levels of inflammation, as can diabetes that is not under control. Obviously, you need to treat these conditions and get them under control. If you're a smoker, then you need to quit smoking to reduce your risk from the inflammation, as well as the spasms caused in your arteries from the by products of smoking. A newly identified culprit of inflammation is periodontal (gum) disease. Studies show that people with moderate to advanced gum disease are almost twice as likely to have a heart attack and about three times as likely to have a stroke. You need to see your dentist, have a periodontal examination and if you have gum disease, get it treated.

Are women more at risk from inflammatory-related heart disease?

Both sexes are at risk so don't kid yourself. Remember, there are no symptoms when you are at risk. Because women have heart attacks that are caused quite often by spasms of the arteries leading to the heart, women of younger ages without evidence of cholesterol plaques may still have heart attacks. Women also have smaller arteries so they get blocked more easily when the vessels spasm, especially if inflammation causes this to happen.

Women who have elevated levels of inflammation on a HS-CRP blood test have a 4 times higher risk of a heart attack than women with normal levels.

Can your dentist really play a role in reducing your risk of heart attack or stroke?

We might not have any other traditional risk factors for heart disease like smoking or obesity but we all have teeth and gums with bacteria. Our gums are coated with a bacterial plaque called a biofilm and thanks to these bacteria, it's estimated that 3 in 4 Americans have some form of gum disease.

According to new findings from Dr. Offenbacher and his team at the University of North Carolina, your dentist could play an important new role in your health care team to help you prevent a sudden, unexpected heart attack or stroke. Here's why:

Studies show that people with gum disease are almost twice as likely to have a heart attack and about 3 times as likely to have a stroke. However, we do know that the more severe the level of gum disease (and 7–15 percent of the adult U.S. population have advanced-stage gum disease), the more severe the thickening of the arteries and the higher the C-reactive protein inflammatory response that is associated with increased risk for heart attack or stroke.

Although we still don't understand all of the causes or inflammatory triggers that actually damage the arteries and ultimately the heart, it now appears that gum disease may be one of the new identifiable causes that we can diagnose, prevent, and treat.

ANOTHER NEW BEST MEASURE FOR HEART RISK: APOB

Move over, cholesterol, there's a new test on the block that some researchers say is even more predictive of heart attack risk. This new best test is called apolipoprotein or Apo for short. Measuring apolipoproteins, tiny fat particles floating in the blood—specifically one type of apolipoprotein, ApoB—signals a high risk of clogged arteries and heart attacks. Some experts would argue that the ratio of ApoB to ApoA1 in the blood is more important in predicting heart risk than the ratio of LDL cholesterol to HDL or good cholesterol.

There are a couple of advantages to measuring ApoB. First, you don't have to be fasting before giving a blood sample as you do with cholesterol tests. Second, ApoB is a better measure of predicting heart risk than LDL in patients taking cholesterol-lowering drugs. But because the measure of cholesterol has been so ingrained in the psyche of both patients and doctors, it will be years before newer tests are understood and accepted. Our advice: Get your doctor to starting ordering ApoB and HSCRP tests now. Why not learn as much as possible about your risk.

HOMOCYSTEINE: AN UNKNOWN RISK FACTOR

Here's something that we're willing to bet you're not aware of, but doctors think you should be. There's a substance in your body that's rarely talked about that has been shown to increase your risk of dying from heart attacks and stroke, people with high levels of it are about three times more at risk compared to persons with low levels. This substance is called **homocysteine**—an amino acid found normally in your body and used to help manufacture protein, a basic building block of muscle.

The trouble starts when you have too high a level of homocysteine in your body. Kidney damage and certain genetic disorders elevate homocysteine. Vitamin deficiency can also cause elevated levels. In healthy individuals, the homocysteine that people normally manufacture is converted into harmless amino acids but requires three B vitamins: B_6, B_{12}, and most important, folate. Folate is the natural form of this essential vitamin but is supplied as folic acid in vitamins and supplements. Most people don't get enough of it because their diets are lacking in green leafy vegetables, grains, and fruits. (Pregnant women should know that folic acid is needed for the proper development of the spinal cord and brain in the developing fetus.) If you have low levels of any these three vitamins, homocysteine levels increase.

Elevated levels of homocysteine are thought to damage arterial walls. The buildup of cholesterol in these scarred arteries leads to the blockages that help produce the increased risk of heart attacks and strokes. There are no formal recommendations telling patients or physicians who should have homocysteine levels tested. Some doctors recommend testing people who have an early family history of narrowing of the arteries or who have cardiovascular disease without other apparent risk factors for this disease.

In the absence of recommendations, here's what many physicians are doing to lower their own levels of homocysteine (and we think you should to):

- Taking a daily multivitamin that provides 100 percent of the RDA of B_6 (4 mg), B_{12} (25 mcg), and folate (400 mcg). Folate or folic acid supplements seem to decrease homocysteine levels more than getting folate strictly via the diet.

- Eating lots of leafy greens, whole grains, fish, and fruits.

More research needs to be done to definitely prove that lowering homocysteine levels alone will be of benefit in reducing the risk of cardiovascular disease, but why take a chance? Doctors know to do this . . . and you should too.

ASPIRIN THERAPY EVERY DAY

Because more Americans die of coronary heart disease (CHD) than from anything else, the U.S. Preventive Services Task Force (USPSTF—a group of national experts representing many different medical groups and organizations, including the government, that come together and recommend what testing should be done on various groups of people and at what ages, based on the latest medical findings) has focused some of its efforts on reducing the rate of heart attacks in the general population. In January 2002, it made a recommendation regarding aspirin therapy in healthy adult patients who were at increased risk for heart disease. Those they considered at increased risk are men older than forty years, postmenopausal women, and younger persons with risk factors for CHD like smoking, high blood pressure, and diabetes. The group found that the regular use of aspirin reduced the risk of CHD by 28 percent in persons who were at increased risk and had never had a heart attack.

There are some problems associated with the regular use of aspirin. It can increase the risk of gastrointestinal or GI bleeding (enteric coated and buffered aspirin do not clearly reduce this). It can also cause a small increase in the incidence of hemorrhagic strokes, i.e., the 20 percent of strokes that cause bleeding inside the brain. The harm may exceed the benefits for those at low risk for CHD, so its best for all persons to discuss the use of aspirin with their doctors. A single baby aspirin is as effective as higher doses.

Aspirin and Bypass Surgery— A New Benefit

While we're on the subject of aspirin, we thought we'd digress for just a minute and slip in the results of some new research that has surprised most doctors. Not only does your doctor need to know about this benefit of aspirin, but you should too.

Previously, it was thought that if a person was given aspirin prior to bypass surgery or immediately after this surgery, they would be at an increased risk of bleeding, which in turn would lead to more complications. This theory was routinely taught to all surgeons and it made sense . . . until this latest research. The new data clearly shows that taking an aspirin either before heart bypass surgery or immediately afterward significantly reduces your risk of dying from heart attacks or strokes. No longer do you have to worry about stopping aspirin prior to bypass surgery. This just applies to bypass surgery and not to other surgeries. It also does not apply if your doctor gives other anticlotting medicines.

Interestingly enough, when you take your daily aspirin can make a difference as well. Researchers in Spain found that taking aspirin at night before going to bed lowered blood pressure in well persons and in those with mild blood pressure problems.

Don't forget that the aspirin has been proven to reduce the risk of future problems in persons who've already had a stroke, a transient ischemic attack or TIA, or a heart attack. If you fall into one of these categories, talk to your doctor about the safety of taking aspirin. The benefit is clear if it doesn't interfere with other medicines.

OMEGA-3 FATTY ACIDS CAN REDUCE YOUR RISK OF HEART ATTACKS

The American Heart Association (AHA) has just released their recommendations on omega-3 fatty acid supplements. It's the first time in history that the AHA has endorsed a supplement to lessen the chances of a heart attack.

Numerous studies have found that consuming as little as one gram a day of omega-3 fatty acids can reduce a person's risk of heart attacks and improve survival rates. Use of omega-3s can reduce a man's risk of heart attack by 50 percent and a woman's by 33 percent. The AHA believes that these are fantastic improvements for very little effort.

Omega-3 fatty acids are found in fish oil from fatty fish. Fish high in omega-3s are salmon, white tuna, mackerel, swordfish, Atlantic char, and trout. These fish can also contain high sources of mercury that can be a concern for pregnant women and young children and should be eaten no more than once a week by these two groups. For other persons, these fish do not warrant concern at this time. Because many people can't eat fish or don't like fish, a supplement containing a gram of omega-3 fatty acids can serve the same purpose.

VITAMIN E AND YOUR HEART

Some studies have shown that vitamin E can lower the risk of heart attack in women by 40 percent and that of men by 35 percent. Vitamin E is a fat-soluble vitamin known as an antioxidant (it slows oxidation in your body). Oxidation causes the cells in your arteries to more easily absorb the "bad" or LDL cholesterol, which promotes plaque formation and the narrowing of arteries. This vitamin is believed to limit the buildup of this dangerous cholesterol in artery walls. If you take 400 IU of vitamin E daily, your cardiovascular system has a better chance of remaining young.

The key to the success of vitamin E is using it before the buildup of plaque in your arteries occurs and before they become permanently hardened. Rarely does a person get enough vitamin E from his or her diet, so supplements are essential.

We should note here that never studies have shown mixed results from high doses of vitamin E. Although some studies clearly show a decrease of heart disease in women who take high-doses of vitamin E, others show no benefit at all. The jury may be out until longer term studies can be done, for the meantime, our advice is to take a vitamin E supplement containing 400 IU per day. The only downside to this is that some patients have an increased risk of bleeding when vitamin E and aspirin are used together. Check with your doctor before taking this combination, especially if you have a risk of ulcers or bleeding disorders.

WHAT DOCTORS WOULD DO ...
And You Should Too

1. If you're over age thirty, take the following supplements on a daily basis:

   - Vitamin E: 400 IU
   - Folic acid: 400 mcg

- B_6: 4 mg
- B_{12}: 25 mcg
- Omega-3 fatty acids: 1 gram

2. Take a baby aspirin daily if not contraindicated by your doctor.

3. Get a C-reactive protein blood test taken. If elevated, address risk factors if present and reduce where possible.

4. Lower your cholesterol and CRP by using statin drugs where appropriate.

RISK FACTORS FOR THE LEADING KILLERS OF WOMEN AND MEN

Nearly 62 million people are estimated to have cardiovascular disease, including about 12 million with coronary artery disease (the arteries leading to the heart). There are two major risk factors for cardiovascular disease that are *not* under our control. These are age and a family history of early heart attack or stroke. All we can do with these two risk factors is be aware of them and pay more attention to those that we can control. We'd like to share some important insights into some key risk factors that will surprise you and provide some information that can make a difference in your risk.

Blood Pressure

About 50 million Americans are estimated to be hypertensive (have an elevated blood pressure). Inadequately controlled blood pressure is one of the biggest risk factors for heart disease, stroke, congestive heart failure and kidney failure due to hypertension. There is no shortage of drugs (nine different classes of blood pressure medicines) or money (12 billion dollars spent in the United States alone) to treat high blood pressure but unfortunately, less than one quarter of persons with hypertension are controlled to the treatment goal of 140/90 mm Hg. As a result, the National Heart, Lung, and Blood Institute of the National Institutes of Health have just issued the 7th report (JNC 7) on U.S. guidelines for the prevention and treatment of hypertension.

The biggest surprise with the new JNC 7 guidelines is the addition of a new category as part of the blood pressure classification scheme: "prehypertension." This includes persons with a systolic blood pressure between 120–139 or a diastolic blood pressure between 80–89. The experts did this for two reasons:

1. Blood pressure increases steadily as we age and most people will develop hypertension during their lifetime. Some data exists that shows even if we have normal blood pressure when we're fifty-five years old, we still have a 90 percent lifetime risk of developing hypertension at some point.

2. Studies show that even at blood pressure levels as low as 115/75 mm Hg there is an increased risk of heart attacks, strokes, and other blood vessel problems. The data further shows that there's as much as a doubling of the risk for cardiovascular death for every 20 mm rise in systolic and 10 mm rise in diastolic in blood pressure above this ideal level.

If you are one of the approximately 46 million people who do fall into this new "prehypertension" category, then experts recommend only lifestyle changes to prevent developing actual hypertension. These changes might include weight reduction, exercise, dietary changes, salt reduction, limiting alcohol intake and of course, not smoking.

Under the new guidelines, there are now only 3 categories for blood pressure: normal systolic (under 120 mm Hg) and diastolic (under 80 mm Hg), prehypertension, and hypertension. Hypertension is defined as anyone with a blood pressure greater than 140/90 for persons with normal health risks. Treatment should begin at this point. If a person has diabetes or chronic kidney disease, then treatment should begin when blood pressure is greater than 130/80.

The bottom line is that hypertension is not being controlled in the majority of people with this problem. As a result, the risk of heart disease, strokes, and heart failure has not been impacted as it should with all the drugs and money we've thrown at it. One of the major reasons for failing to control blood pressure is poor patient compliance. It's important that you familiarize yourself with the new blood pressure guidelines and that you take the medication your doctor prescribes. If you have problems with your medication, work with your doctor to reduce side effects. Discuss the possibility of using low-dose combination drug therapies or convenient dosing like once-a-day medications. If your physician hasn't involved you in your treatment by the use of home blood pressure monitoring, ask him or her to do so. If your doctor won't teach you how to do this or isn't interested, it's time to get another doctor.

Cholesterol

Problems with cholesterol (dyslipidemia is the medical name for this) are one of the most important of the modifiable risk factors for coronary heart disease. Cholesterol in and of itself is not bad. Indeed, it is so essential to the health of the cells within our bodies that we make it naturally. Our liver makes 80 percent of the cholesterol that our body needs. Our diets clearly impact the levels of cholesterol in our bodies, but to a lesser degree than many people believe. Even if we could possibly eat no cholesterol, our cholesterol levels would still remain well above zero since our body manufactures so much of it naturally.

The problems start when we have too much cholesterol. And the biggest problem here is that most people with elevated cholesterol or hyperlipidemia are not receiving proper treatment. Of the estimated 8 million people with cholesterol problems, only about one-quarter have received diet therapy and only about 10 percent of eligible people are getting drug therapy . . . and you can't blame lack of insurance for this undertreatment. In one study of managed care health plan enrollees, only one-third of those who should have been receiving therapy for elevated cholesterol were actually being treated. The other problem: Only about half of those receiving treatment to reduce their LDL or bad cholesterol were receiving adequate treatment. These study results indicate a major problem in our health care system and its ability to lower one risk associated with heart disease. Doctors are just not being aggressive enough about reducing cholesterol levels. Even when correctly treated by their doctors, many people are not getting proper therapy. Why? Noncompliance on the part of patients—they're just not taking their medication or following the diet prescribed to them. This is something we just don't understand when reduced cholesterol is so vital to your health.

What are some other reasons for reducing cholesterol levels? Women can reduce their risk of dying from a clot related stroke by almost 25 percent by getting their cholesterol back to normal. African-American women can cut their risk by 50 percent or more over a lifetime by treating high cholesterol. New research also shows that high cholesterol levels may double a person's risk of developing Alzheimer's disease. Do you need any more reasons?

The Good, the Bad, and the Ugly Cholesterol

Understanding your cholesterol and its potential impact on your health means more than just knowing a single number like your total cholesterol. This one test is fine for a rough screening, but not sufficient for truly evaluating your risk of heart disease or stroke. If all your doctor is measuring is your total cholesterol and basing his or her treatment on this, find another doctor. Assessment of your cholesterol health requires an evaluation of your HDL, LDL, and triglycerides as well. It would be comparable to your dentist only taking a superficial look at your teeth and never taking X rays of your mouth, or your car mechanic checking your oil and none of the other important parts of your engine and then stating that all looks well. A complete evaluation of your cholesterol requires an understanding of three other lipids in order to put the entire cholesterol picture into better focus. Here they are:

The Good: HDL (high-density lipoprotein); carries artery-clogging cholesterol away from the arteries to the liver for breakdown. Levels of HDL can be raised by exercise and red wine. Levels of HDL greater than 60 mg/dL are generally protective against heart disease while levels below 40 are a risk factor.

The Bad: LDL (low-density lipoprotein); helps promote the buildup of plaque in artery walls. High LDL levels put a person at considerable risk for heart attacks and strokes. Ideal levels should be 130 mg/dL or below.

The Ugly: Your triglycerides (fatty substances in the blood); cholesterol levels can be normal, but if triglycerides are high, people may be at considerable risk for cardiovascular disease. Levels should be kept under 200 mg/dL.

What the best doctors have come to know and to believe is that lipid-lowering therapy with drugs like the statins may stabilize cholesterol plaques in the arteries and at the same time lower the risk of thrombus or blockage in the heart. Such treatment might also reduce the risk of coronary events or heart attacks by reducing the inflammation thought to be associated with them. The statin class of drugs may actually provide a double benefit.

New Cholesterol Guidelines

The National Cholesterol Education Program (NCEP) has issued three sets of guidelines to treat high blood cholesterol through its Adult Treatment Panel (ATP I, ATP II, and ATP III). The first set of guidelines focused on long-term primary prevention of cholesterol by diet, while ATP II emphasized secondary prevention with diet and cholesterol-lowering drugs in patients with coronary heart disease. The new guidelines set forth in ATP III were published in 2001 and provide a quantitative estimate of a person's ten-year risk of myocardial infarction (heart attack) or coronary death. Based on this system, if a patient's risk is above 10 percent they are considered to be at moderately high risk for coronary heart disease (CHD). If you have these risks, many doctors now strongly believe that you should undergo primary preventive therapy. You can get your own risk assessment using the Framingham Points Scale by going to www.nhlbi.nih.gov/guidelines/cholesterol/index.htm.

By using the scoring system, ATP III greatly expands secondary prevention, but most important, it increases the number of patients eligible for aggressive cholesterol-lowering therapy. For the first time ever, not only is it recommended that persons with established heart disease be treated, but also those who have an equivalent risk based on risk factors.

Physicians are a big part of the problem. The guidelines for treating elevated cholesterol in patients at risk or those with equivalent risk are very clear. Even though ATP I and ATP II have been out for years, less than 25 percent of people who require treatment for cholesterol are being treated properly. Failure of physicians to treat according to the NCEP guidelines is the biggest reason patients are at increased risk for cardiovascular disease from cholesterol-related causes. Obviously, as we stated earlier, part of the problem lies with patients not being compliant with treatment. One study showed that better than 30 percent of patients who were put on cholesterol-lowering drugs actually took them. We've got no one to blame but ourselves when this happens.

Our advice to you: Don't wait on your doctor to determine your risk and suggest treatment. First, get all the cholesterol measurements we mentioned above, and then take the Framingham Points Scale test for yourself. If your score is below 10, you are at low risk for heart problems. If above 20, you are at high risk and you should see your doctor because treatment is strongly recommended. Obviously, if your HDL cholesterol is low or your LDL and/or triglycerides are high, you should already be under treatment, beginning with diet therapy and followed by drug therapy if diet doesn't bring about the necessary changes (and frankly, it's not likely to). Increasing physical activity and getting your weight under control are the cornerstones of good cholesterol treatment as well.

One thing we all have to remember, lowering our cholesterol, like reducing many of our risk factors, is a preventive measure and the benefit may not be seen for years. It's easy to focus our efforts on a medical problem when we are ill. How many people vow to start exercising, to eat properly, and to stop smoking immediately after a heart attack? Almost everyone does because they're extremely scared and think they're going to die. But what do we see happening all too frequently a few weeks later? When the person begins feeling better again, the good intentions go right out the window. Now just imagine how difficult it is to get someone to eat properly, take medicines daily, and perform other healthy behaviors when they feel fine. This is the dilemma that we face with cholesterol. Are you up to the challenge?

THE DIABETES EPIDEMIC AND HEART DISEASE

Diabetes is epidemic and it's getting worse by the year. It's estimated that 17 million Americans have the disease but almost 40 percent of them have *not* been diagnosed. There are two types of diabetes. Type 1 occurs most often during childhood or adolescence and accounts for up to 10 percent of the cases. Type 2 occurs most commonly in persons older than forty and represents almost 90 percent of cases. Diabetes is a major risk factor for heart disease and stroke.

Insulin is made in the pancreas and is needed to drive glucose or sugar into the body's cells, where it can be utilized for energy purposes. In diabetics, the body either stops making insulin or doesn't make enough, so the glucose in the blood builds up. In recent years, researchers have become aware of a relationship between insulin resistance syndrome and atherosclerosis. Patients who are diabetic are at tremendous risk for blood-vessel-related problems. Eighty percent of diabetic patients die because of coronary atherosclerosis (cholesterol plaque in the arteries of the heart) and/or peripheral vascular disease (blockage of the arteries in the extremities, primarily the legs).

There are two principal reasons for this epidemic of diabetes: obesity and aging. When people become obese, they become resistant to insulin so it doesn't work as well to do its primary job—lowering blood sugar levels. More and more of our kids are obese today thanks to a lack of physical activity caused in part by video games and an excessive time spent in chairs in front of computers. It's this extra weight that causes the insulin resistance that creates heart disease, and this is why we have more type-1 diabetics today. Hispanics and African-Americans have the highest percentage of new diabetics in our population, most of this is due to increasing numbers of young people being obese.

The other reason for the increase in diabetes cases is aging. As persons get older, the beta cells in their pancreas (the place where insulin is made) fail. When they produce less insulin, sugar builds up in our systems and we develop diabetes as an adult—type 2 diabetes.

A number of medications can be used to treat diabetes, but this is entirely beyond the scope of this book. So what can we do to reduce our risk of diabetes and delay the need to take medications? There are a couple of things doctors know to do:

See a nutritionist a few times to control diet: Consulting a person skilled in nutrition clearly improves the control of blood sugars and reduces the need for medications.

Get off the couch and begin exercising: Exercise helps to burn calories and reduce our blood sugars so that we need less insulin. It also helps to reduce our weight and this means less resistance to insulin. Many type 2 diabetics can be controlled for many years by something as simple as walking regularly and keeping their weight under control.

Diabetes is one of the most important risk factors for heart disease not to mention kidney disease, stroke, eye disease (called diabetic retinopathy), and neurologic or nerve problems. If you are diabetic, you should be receiving regular examinations of other parts of your body to check for complications. Here are some things that your doctor should be checking for annually if not more often:

Skin examinations of the lower extremities: Diabetics lose the sensory feeling in their feet as a result of nerve damage. They get skin breakdown, ulcers, and nonhealing wounds. If undetected, severe problems, which can result in the loss of an extremity, can occur.

Eye examinations: Diabetics develop problems with their retina deep within the eye. If not treated early, loss of vision can be the ultimate outcome.

Specialized blood testing called a Hemoglobin A1C: This provides doctors with a sense of a person's overall blood sugar levels. Hemoglobin A1C levels should be kept below 7 percent.

Blood tests for kidney function and lipids: Diabetics are at considerable risk for kidney and lipid (cholesterol) disorders. If not detected early, these can put a person at severe risk for heart disease and stroke, and if kidney function decreases, they may require a kidney transplant or dialysis.

If you're diabetic and you're not getting the above examinations at least yearly, get to another doctor. We cannot emphasize enough the need to be screened regularly for this disease, especially if you have a family history of diabetes or you are overweight. It's just too important to your long-term health not to be aware and be checked.

UNDERUSE OF PROVEN THERAPIES IN HEART DISEASE

Physicians find it extremely difficult to maintain clinical competence when faced with the demands of a busy practice and the constant advances in medical knowledge. Believe it or not, many doctors often treat patients the exact same way that they learned when in residency training . . . and this could have been ten or twenty years earlier. Can you imagine going to a mechanic who treated modern-day cars in the same manner as he did a car twenty years ago? Could you imagine an athlete today not taking advantage of modern technology and instead using equipment that was developed ten or more years ago? We think not.

Unfortunately, many physicians are practicing "old-style" medicine and not taking advantage of the latest research. Here are a few facts that may shock you:

■ Despite the overwhelming benefit of a class of drugs called beta-blockers in the treatment of heart failure, only about 10 percent of heart failure patients are prescribed such drugs.

■ Following a heart attack, these same beta-blockers have been proven to reduce both complications and death if given at the time of discharge. Unfortunately, studies show that doctors prescribe the medicine in only about one-third of patients in the best studies and around 10 percent in studies with the worst results.

■ Patients with high blood pressure have their blood pressure under proper control only about 50 percent of the time because many doctors aren't following treatment guidelines set forth by national organizations such as the National Institute of Health.

■ Only 30 percent of patients with heart failure are given the appropriate medicine for treating their condition. (It should be an angiotensin-converting enzyme (ACE) inhibitor in most cases.)

■ Eighty-four percent of diabetic patients did not receive blood tests for hemoglobin A1C to monitor the control of their diabetes.

■ Only 18 percent of patients with known heart disease and 40 percent of persons at high risk for it had their LDL or bad cholesterol under control.

Have we gotten your attention yet? The point we're trying to make is that too many people are not receiving optimal medical care because their doctors do not follow the most up-to-date medical guidelines. And it's not necessarily the case that these are bad doctors; even the best-intentioned doctors have a difficult time keeping up with the latest therapies. So what can you do? Educate yourself. Make it a point to research your own medical condition. It's relatively easy today to find numerous Web sites that provide excellent patient education. You can't always count on your doctor being up on the latest therapies, even in a condition as common as heart disease. Just imagine what could happen with a less common medical disease. Why take a chance? Be your own advocate; do the research, ask the questions, and make sure you're getting the best medical care available.

EBCT SCANNING FOR HEART DISEASE: HOLD ON TO YOUR WALLET

EBCT (electron beam computed tomography) scanning is a form of computed tomography that is also known as ultrafast CT scanning or coronary calcium screening. It is used to detect calcium deposits in the arteries of your heart. Why is this important? The coronary arteries supply blood to the heart and they are considered diseased when cholesterol plaque accumulates in the walls of the arteries. The medical term for this condition is atherosclerosis. These plaques are initially made of soft cholesterol. Over time, the cholesterol in the arteries can become calcified, but not always, and that's part of the problem and why there's so much controversy associated with the EBCT test.

EBCT is designed to measure the amount of calcium in the coronary arteries, but just finding calcium in the coronary arteries doesn't mean much. Because of our high-fat diets (especially our predeliction for fast food), nearly everyone over twenty-five has some calcium in their arteries. But these calcium deposits aren't necessarily significant to your health. Just having them doesn't mean you are going to develop heart disease. You will need more tests to determine its true significance. But proponents of EBCT believe that a positive test can get people to change their habits before things get worse. The data in smokers with positive chest X rays does not indicate this to be true. So are EBCTs a good idea or not?

Here's the rest of the problem. If EBCT shows your arteries are free of calcium, it doesn't mean that you are free of heart disease. You may have significant plaque that's accumulated in your artery walls and is producing blockage, but unless it's calcified, you'll never see it on the EBCT. You'll come away from the test feeling like you've gotten a clean bill of health when it fact you haven't.

Now that we know more about the test, what's the real issue here? Why do you even care? Well, here's what's happening that's of concern to many doctors (we agree and that's why we're including this section in the book). Local clinics are now advertising EBCT tests directly to the public: "Come on down and get a quick scan over your lunch break to find out if you're at risk for heart disease." The advertisements and brochures advocating EBCT often target the worried well—people who are healthy and have no known risk factors for heart disease. These clinics make outlandish claims of how EBCT can save your life, and people who are worried about heart disease come running.

EBCT centers do *not* require a referral from your doctor and will cost you an average of five hundred dollars for this twenty-minute scan. Most insurers will *not* cover the cost of these tests unless ordered by a doctor for a specific clinical indication. So is this test worth it? We think not, and most doctors agree.

Many doctors do not think EBCT is a good idea and it's simply a moneymaking ploy on the part of those advocating it. It's a test that's been around for twenty years yet it's still not accepted for widespread use. The American College of Cardiology and the American Heart Association issued a joint opinion on EBCT in 2000 that concludes that EBCT should not be used in routine clinical practice or to screen patients who have no symptoms. Need we say more?

Until there is more evidence based on good clinical trials, we advise you not to use EBCT unless ordered by a doctor for a specific clinical indication. It can be useful in following the progression of heart disease in some people and in people with specific known risk factors for heart disease. EBCT should not be used in people who've already had a heart attack, (because of the damage in their hearts, test results cannot be read as well); people who have undergone coronary bypass surgery or angioplasty; and women who are pregnant (because of the high amount of radiation two test puts out). What doctors know and you should too . . . see your doctor for a workup before heading for an EBCT. It will save you time, money, and further unneeded testing.

HORMONE THERAPY, HEART DISEASE, AND CANCER RISK: OUR TAKE ON IT ALL

How could we write a chapter on important cardiovascular health issues and not talk about hormone replacement therapy (HRT) in women? Remember, for many years menopausal women were placed on hormones to reduce their risk of heart disease. What we know now is that the use of HRT to reduce the risk of heart disease in women is unwarranted. In 2002, the NIH-sponsored hormone therapy trial results were announced three years earlier than expected. The trial, known as the Women's Health Initiative (WHI), was stopped prematurely because the results indicated an increased health risk for women who took hormones. There's been a great deal of controversy and confusion over the results of the WHI, so we thought we'd try to make them a bit clearer for you so that you can make your own decisions armed with the facts and in consultation with your own doctor.

Here's why the study was stopped. Women's Health Initiative researchers came to the conclusion that taking estrogen plus progestin increases the risks of heart disease, breast cancer, and other problems. Women on hormones had more heart attacks, breast cancer, colon cancer, blood clots, and strokes than women who took a placebo (sugar pills). The heart disease risk occurred in the first year of treatment, while the other risks increased with time. Before the results of this study, conventional theory held that women on HRT reduced their risk of heart disease and stroke because normal levels of estrogen protected women from cardiovascular disease. The WHI study shot this theory full of holes (see table below).

Hormone Therapy Trial Results

	Hormone Replacement Group*	Placebo Group*
Heart Attack	37	30
Stroke	29	21
Blood Clots	34	16
Breast Cancer	38	30
Colon Cancer	10	16
Fractures	10	15

*Yearly cases per 10,000 women
Source: Women's Health Initiative

It's hard to argue with the data, but many have tried. Controversy surrounded the findings when they first came out. Doctors felt blindsided by the news. It was totally unexpected news and against all they'd been taught. The WHI researchers quickly moved to make sense out of the findings for women and debunk the critics. Many women didn't wait for the scientists to sort out things, but got off hormones. Sales of the hormone Prempro dropped 30 percent immediately after the results were announced.

What women quickly discovered when they went off hormones (and we heard from many of them on our Speaking of Women's Health Tour) was that the symptoms that drove them crazy and made them go on hormones in the first place came right back. Women complained of hot flashes, insomnia, mood changes, and general irritability. (We heard of many husbands who wished that their wives would go back on hormones as soon as possible.) Tapering off hormones slowly helped some women to avoid withdrawal problems, while others used antidepressants to reduce hot flashes and sweats. Some women found that eliminating spicy foods and avoiding caffeine helped. A great many found that nothing seemed to help them like the hormones did. Many women were now caught in a quandary. Should they take a potential risk with their future to achieve a benefit in the quality of their life now? It's not an easy answer.

Recent data from a study on the use of hormones to reduce the risk of Alzheimer's disease adds more fuel to the fiery debate. Women who had used hormones were 40 percent less likely to develop Alzheimer's than those who never used them. There were two problems with this data. Women who showed this benefit had taken hormones for more than ten years, and they decided to do this on their own rather than being in a controlled study. Until a more scientific study is done, these results should not be used as a basis for putting women on hormones to reduce the risk of Alzheimer's disease. Here's our advice: Speak to your doctor to best put your potential risk into perspective. Only then can you decide the benefits that HRT can bring to your ability to function day to day.

What Should Women Do Now?

Here are the current recommendations regarding HRT that most doctors would agree upon:

- Nobody should take HRT for long-term protection against chronic diseases.

- Going on hormones to protect against heart disease is unwarranted.

- For relief of the symptoms of menopause, women who want to use hormones should try the smallest dose for the shortest period possible.

What Women Can Do to Prevent Their Risk of Getting a Heart Attack

1. **Don't Smoke:** Cigarettes significantly increase the odds of a heart attack. What women don't realize is that smoking increases a woman's risk of heart disease more than a man's.

2. **Exercise Is the Best Defense:** Next to not smoking, this is the most important thing that you can do. New guidelines from the National Institutes of Medicine recommend sixty minutes of activity per day. But if that isn't realistic for you, don't despair. Even walking or exercising for ten-minute stretches a few times a day will get you there painlessly. A little exercise is better than nothing at all.

3. **Two Drinks a Day Can Protect Your Heart:** Here's some advice that is easier to follow than point number two. Two drinks a day has been shown to reduce a woman's risk of heart disease even more than not drinking alcohol at all. Caution: The benefits fall off if you drink more than this.

4. **Women Need to Know Their Numbers:** Even cholesterol testing is different for women than it is for men. Whereas high levels of LDL, the so-called bad cholesterol, are helpful in identifying men at high risk of heart disease, women are more vulnerable to high levels of a different fatty substance, called triglycerides. Also, thanks to natural estrogen, women usually have high levels of HDL or good cholesterol. If a woman happens to have low levels of HDL, she is more likely than a man to develop heart disease. National guidelines suggest a minimum HDL level of 40 mg/dL for men and women. But since low HDL is a more powerful predictor of risk in women, many doctors now recommend keeping an HDL of 50 mg/dL for women. Make sure to talk to your doctor about your numbers at your next checkup.

5. **What You Eat Matters . . . A Lot:** Fewer than one in four Americans gets the recommended five or more servings of greens, vegetables, and other heart-healthy produce. Why does this matter? Because there are phytochemicals in spinach, tomatoes, and carrots, to name a few, that help protect against heart disease. A healthy diet can protect your heart and your health.

6. **Relax:** Stress affects women more significantly than it affects men. And researchers have found that there is a clear link between heart disease and stress. So give yourself a break and do something fun every day. It's the best medicine you can give yourself.

- Women taking hormones to prevent osteoporosis should consider switching to other drugs for that purpose. A bone density test can help show if newer medications called biphosphonates can be of benefit.

- If vaginal dryness is your primary concern, there are several good nonprescription, nonhormonal creams like Astroglide and Replens that can be helpful.

There are still many, many unanswered questions about hormone use in women with menopause symptoms, especially about which particular subgroup of women may be at greatest risk. Is estrogen alone safe to use since it increases the risk of uterine cancer? Who should use hormones and for how long to relieve the symptoms of menopause and still be safe? Studies are now under way to answer these and other questions. For now, women will have to carefully weigh the risks and the benefits before continuing on hormones.

Summary

The field of cardiovascular medicine is changing constantly as more studies of large populations are done and we learn more about the impact of various therapies on long-term health. Patients need to constantly educate themselves about these studies and do the appropriate research on the Internet about their particular medical condition. Cardiovascular disease is the number one killer in the U.S. Doctors know that they need to monitor their own condition and be aggressive in their therapy . . . and you should too.

CHAPTER NINE

CANCER AND CANCER SCREENING: WHAT YOU DON'T KNOW COULD KILL YOU

What if we told you that we could help you reduce your risk of getting or dying from the disease women and men fear the most? The answer is a no-brainer. Trust us. This is not just hype. The information that we provide in this chapter can truly help you reduce your risk of cancer.

When we're out talking with people in our speeches and seminars or when we're taking care of patients in our clinical practices, it almost always surprises them to learn that Cancer is *not* the number one killer in the United States, nor is it the underlying cause of death in a majority of people. However, it is one of the most feared diseases that people can get because of the often painful, slow way we see many cancer victims die. In fact, in a recent Harris poll, 67 percent of women listed cancer as their number one fear. We also know that patients fear cancer because of the effects of radiation and/or chemotherapy. Let's shed some light on cancer and see if we can help put you more in control. Some of what we may talk about in this chapter may be a little technical and there may be a few more statistics than usual, but this will help you to better understand why we make certain recommendations (it also may be good ammunition for your doctor, as he may not be aware of some of this information either).

WHAT'S CANCER?

Cancer is not one disease but rather numerous diseases characterized by abnormal cells that divide uncontrollably and invade normal body tissue. But all cancers share a common origin. Cancers are caused by genetic mutations (changes in our DNA at the cellular level), either inherited or acquired, that ultimately result in abnormal cells being formed that progress to cancer over time. Cancer often forms tumors (a mass of abnormal cells) that invades or impairs normal tissues. Not all tumors are cancerous, and not all cancers form tumors. Some cancers occur in the bone marrow and cause the disease we know as leukemia. We also know that cancer takes a while to develop and that cancers may be in our bodies for years before we begin to develop their signs or symptoms.

Unfortunately, there are many myths and misconceptions associated with cancer prevention and screening. One of these is that all cancer screening is painful, and another is that such screening doesn't do any good because many of us know people who were screened but still developed cancer. (Neither of these is true, by the way.) Such myths contribute to unnecessary deaths because men and women fail to get the proper care, screening, and treatment. Another myth is that regular checkups and today's advanced medical technology can detect all cancer early. As you'll read later on, regular medical care can increase your chances of detecting cancer early, but it's no guarantee. And, until a cancer grows to a certain size, there is no existing technology that is capable of detecting it.

And let's not discount the fear factor. Some people may not want to go for a cancer screening out of fear that the doctor will find something. But early detection is often the key to survival. So please, if there's one message that we want to get across to you, it's the need to get going and get screened.

Learn what doctors know about screening so that you can increase your chances of beating cancer if it should come your way. Your greatest risk is not knowing. With cancer, it's what you don't know that can kill you. We think you'll agree when you finish this chapter.

CANCER SCREENING

The best cancer screening tools detect abnormal cells before they become cancerous or detect cancers in their early stages so they can be removed before they cause serious problems.

There's an underlying principle of cancer screening that most people, and many physicians, simply don't understand. Just because you can perform a test to find cancer doesn't make that test a good screening tool. There are several characteristics that make a test a good cancer screening method. U.S. health experts have agreed on the following:

- The screening test must detect a cancerous or precancerous condition at a stage when it can still be treated.

- There must be a low false-negative rate—in other words, the test doesn't miss persons who truly have the disease.

- The rate of false-positives must be low so people who really don't have the disease don't undergo unnecessary follow-up procedures and treatments.

- The test must return the same results each time it's given.

- The test must be relatively inexpensive.

- The test should save lives (reduce mortality from the disease).

- The test must be available to large segments of the population.

Ideally, a good screening test should detect disease in an early, asymptomatic stage for the purpose of initiating early intervention and improving the patient's long-term outcome. Later in this chapter, we'll review four types of cancer and the kinds of screening tests that are useful for detecting them. Some of these cancers affect women, some men, and one affects both. (Also see Chapter 3 for more information on tests and when to give them.)

Many currently available tests fail to match many of these criteria. They may miss people who actually have the disease. (Pap tests are a good example of this, if they are not done correctly.) Tests can be too expensive (total body scans) or they don't reduce the death rate from cancer by the time a cancer is found (chest X rays find lung cancers, but it's too late by then).

The United States Preventive Services Task Force (USPSTF) has revised their criteria in the past year for assessing evidence for or against recommending screening tests or procedures during regular health examinations (www.ahrq.gov/clinic/3rduspstf/ratings.htm). Many traditional tests have not been included in those recommendations because they do not meet many of the above criteria. Before any screening is undertaken, the good must outweigh the bad. Not only is the National Cancer Institute (NCI) a good place to research the cancer screening tests that are current and best, but the USPSTF Web site is also a smart place to keep on your radar screen.

One key point that is usually made about cancer screening, and is often touted by its advocates, is that preventive services reduce health care costs. This is *not* true. The data for breast and cervical cancer screening show that the costs of screening tests, the diagnostic follow-up, and the treatment are much higher than the savings in treatment costs. Why is this important to know? Because if you follow the recommendations that we and others make on aggressively screening for certain cancers, you will find some managed care organizations don't cover their costs. Be prepared for this and explore the cancer screening that's allowed under any health plan you're considering before you sign up. If you ask most men and woman, they'll say they're not concerned about the cost, but about preventing and detecting cancer. It might take a few dollars out of your pocket to get the best possible care, but isn't your life worth it?

In 2002, the *Journal of the American Medical Association (JAMA)* published a report that highlighted another fact about cancer that should concern both doctors and patients. African-American patients have a significantly lower survival rate at the end of five years than do white patients. "Numerous studies have demonstrated that blacks are less likely to receive optimal care for cancer than whites and are also more likely to be diagnosed initially at an advanced stage of disease." So what does this mean for you if you're an African-American? African-Americans need to take charge of their health and learn what cancer screening tests should be done and when. Don't wait for a health care provider to tell you. You take charge and insist on the right test at the right time.

TEN KEY FACTS DOCTORS KNOW ABOUT
Cancer and Cancer Prevention . . .
That Most of Us Don't

1. **The earlier most cancers are detected, the better the chances of successfully treating it:** We know that this seems like common sense, but if most women and men know it, why aren't more people getting the kind of cancer screening that they need?

2. **Cancer screening tests are only as good as the health care professional performing the test and/or interpreting the results:** Good doctors know how to perform tests properly and they know the importance of working with a good lab or good radiologist. The key is knowing where your doctor would get her tests performed.

3. **Certain risk factors increase the chances of a person developing specific cancers:** Risk factors vary from cancer to cancer. Some are more important than others. Altering these key risk factors can definitely reduce your chances of getting cancer.

4. **Good cancer screening can markedly reduce your chances of dying from certain kinds of cancer:** Screening tests work to catch cancer early. Some tests are better than others. We'll outline the best tests for you for four key cancers.

5. **Not all doctors follow guidelines or good clinical practice for cancer detection, or for follow-up of abnormal screening test results:** There are definite tests that should be done if abnormalities are found on cancer screening tests. We'll explain what should happen and where you can go to get the most up-to-date information.

6. **Many screening tests for early cancer detection have some flaws, so relying on a single test for assurance is not always a good strategy:** Pap smears, PSA blood tests, and mammograms are not perfect screening tests so medical experts urge frequent repeat testing to ensure early detection of cancer

7. **The follow-up to positive cancer screening test results is not without further risk to your health, and can be very expensive:** There are a certain number of false-positive tests with any screening test. Follow-up on abnormal tests is essential and can create further problems like infection, pain, or unneeded medicines.

8. **Educate yourself on prevention guidelines and on your specific risk factors. Don't rely on others:** Take charge of your own health. Do your research. It's too important to let someone else make these decisions. Some health care providers may not be aware of the latest recommendations.

9. **Preventive screening does not necessarily reduce health care costs:** Medical testing is expensive, and just because a test can be done doesn't make it cost-effective to have it done. Some tests are recommended as first-line tests, with more expensive and more technology-dependent tests saved for later in the screening process.

10. **Not all cancers have good screening tests associated with them:** Some cancers do not lend them themselves to early screening. A screening technology that meets the screening criteria listed above does not currently exist for ovarian or lung cancer, among others. Maybe one day there will such a test, but it's not available at this time.

OBESITY AND THE LINK TO CANCER DEATH

Before we review four cancers in which screening tests have proven beneficial, we want to alert you to some recent findings about cancer. This information can greatly reduce your chances of getting the disease.

In 2003, an American Cancer Society study offered the strongest evidence yet that being overweight increased a person's chances of dying from cancer. The researchers suggested that as many as ninety thousand cancer deaths per year may be related to obesity and could be prevented. The ACS study found that 14 percent of all cancer deaths among men and 20 percent of all cancer deaths in women were associated with being overweight or obese.

Behind tobacco, obesity may be the most important cause of cancer in the United States. The data confirmed the link between excess body weight and breast and colorectal cancer, but also identified a connection between obesity and other cancers not previously linked to it, like stomach cancer and prostate cancer in men, multiple myeloma, non-Hodgkin's lymphoma, and cancers of the cervix, ovary, liver, and pancreas. The message is very clear: Keep your weight under control if you want to reduce your chances of getting cancer.

We will now focus on four major cancers that have adequate screening tests: breast cancer, cervical cancer, colon cancer, and prostate cancer. We know there may be other cancers that may concern you, but none of them—except skin cancer—have good screening tests. There are many good books out there that deal with other cancers and several reputable Web sites that we list at the end of this chapter.

BREAST CANCER

What woman doesn't fear developing breast cancer? Who doesn't know another woman who's been touched by this disease? Who hasn't seen numerous stories in magazines or on television talking about one woman's unique fight with breast cancer? What are the real facts and what can you do about them? Let's look at some information you should know as well as some things that you can do to reduce your risk.

The risk of a woman developing breast cancer over a lifetime is one in every eight women. An average forty-year-old woman's risk of developing breast cancer in the next ten years is less than one in sixty. For an average seventy-year-old woman, the risk increases to about one in twenty-five.

Deaths from breast cancer are second only to lung cancer in all cancer deaths in the United States. In 2002, an estimated forty-thousand women died from breast cancer compared to almost sixty-six thousand who died from lung cancer. (You've come a long way, baby, and it's almost all thanks to smoking!) The good news is that huge advances have been made in the last twenty years in both the treatment and diagnosis of breast cancer. Death from breast cancer has declined by almost 30 percent since 1990 in the United States and Great Britain.

More women die of cardiovascular diseases like heart attack and stroke than all other medical problems put together, but women fear breast cancer more than any other disease. Perhaps it's the disfigurement that surgery can produce, or the underlying fear of recurrence that hangs over any women who've ever had breast

> " The risk of a woman developing breast cancer over a lifetime is one in every eight women. "

cancer, or maybe it's the painful death from cancer that many women have observed in their friends. Maybe it's the media attention given certain cancers (breast being number one). Women need to keep things in perspective. For the average women presently free of breast cancer, the true chance of dying from the disease within the next ten years is extremely small.

What's Your Risk?

You know what most surprises us as we speak to different groups of women? Despite all the educational efforts to date, various studies have found that the majority of them have limited knowledge of the risk factors associated with breast cancer. Two-thirds of the women in one study did not know the importance of age as a risk factor despite the fact that it is the most important one.

Knowledge of risk factors is especially important for women who have first-degree relatives (FDR) with breast cancer. Just having this one risk factor increases a woman's risk of breast cancer by 60 to 80 percent. This risk is increased if the FDR is young or has bilateral disease, or when two or more family members are affected. Unfortunately, the harsh reality is that the majority of breast cancer cases occur in women with no known family history. The point to take home here is that if you have an FDR who's had breast cancer, you need to be even more vigilant and get screenings at an earlier age. If you don't have an FDR with breast cancer, you have a minimal risk for breast cancer unless you have one or more of the risk factors listed below.

It's important to be aware of the factors that can increase your risk:

> "...the majority of breast cancer cases occur in women with no known family history."

- Having had breast cancer once before

- Late age at first pregnancy—having children after the age of thirty

■ Early onset of menstruation—before the age of twelve

■ Having a family history of breast cancer

■ Advanced age

■ Having had a breast biopsy

■ Late onset of menopause.

■ Women who've had radiation to their chests

The more risks you have, the greater the chance of breast cancer, so please be more fastidious about performing breast self-examination (see more about this controversial practice later) and getting annual clinical exams and mammograms. Obviously, as you age, your risk of breast cancer increases, so you need to be more faithful about annual mammograms as you get older.

Women whose breasts appear dense on X ray also seem to be at increased risk for breast cancer. Dense breasts on X ray? What's that mean? It simply means that you happen to have multiple glands and ligaments in your breast tissue plus you don't have much fatty tissue. This is what makes your breasts look denser on an X ray or mammogram. Behavioral factors, like hormone use and alcohol intake, as well as age, can affect density. (We know that you're all sitting there and reading this with a cup of coffee in your hands, and now you're wondering if caffeine can contribute to an increased risk of breast cancer. Let us assure you it does *not*.)

One other disturbing statistic is that black women are more likely to die from breast cancer than white women, even though more cancers are detected in white women. The biggest reasons for this is that mammogram screening rates for black women are much lower.

Is Stress a Risk Factor for Breast Cancer?

One of the concerns women often have—and it springs from the media's intense focus on the subject of breast cancer—is whether stress, emotional upset, personality, or attitude can cause breast cancer or cause it to recur. These concerns are entirely unwarranted: there is no evidence that any of these factors cause breast cancer.

How widespread is this misconception? A recent study in *Psycho-Oncology* reported that 42 percent of women who had survived breast cancer for at least two years believed stress was to blame for their cancer. Further down on the list, 26 percent blamed genetic factors and 25 percent blamed the environment.

The study asked physicians to reexamine how they discussed breast cancer with their patients. The researchers suggested that physicians should ask women what they think the cause of their breast cancer was, and then review the real risk factors with them. We would have to believe that most women with breast cancer (and those who don't have it) would be relieved to know that their emotions did not contribute to their risk of developing the disease.

Genetic Testing and Breast and Ovarian Cancer Risk

Advances in DNA testing have also advanced our understanding of women who are at increased risk for breast cancer. Those women with a specific gene mutation called BRCA1 and BRCA2 have a lifetime risk of breast cancer approaching 70 percent. It's important to note that inherited mutations like these account for only about 10 percent of all breast cancer cases. Mutations in the BRCA genes seem to put women at increased risk for ovarian cancer as well (see table below). Knowing that you are a carrier will help you discuss some serious lifesaving decisions with your doctor.

One study showed that women who tested positive for one of these genes, and then had their ovaries and fallopian tubes removed, lowered their risk of breast and ovarian cancers by 75 percent. Some women with these genetic findings who also have relatives with breast cancer are having their breasts removed ahead of time even without evidence of disease. Preventive double mastectomies like this cut their breast cancer risk by 90 percent. There is much controversy about this radical approach, but it certainly reduces anxiety in those women and almost completely removes the source of potential cancer before it can spread outside the breast. This is a very personal decision and should be made only after getting a couple of opinions from physicians who specialize in breast cancer—medical oncologists. We know one woman who took this approach and she said that it was for two reasons: One, she saw her mother die of breast cancer, and two, she wanted to increase her chances of being around to see her children grow up. We sure couldn't argue with those reasons and we had to admire her courage in making an extremely difficult decision.

Breast and Ovarian Cancer Risk for Women

Population	Breast Cancer Rate	Ovarian Cancer Rate
General population	13%	1.7%
BRCA gene mutation	36% to 85%	16% to 60%

Clearly, having the BRCA gene mutation puts women at considerable increased risk for breast and ovarian cancer. Genetic testing is not something the experts advise for women at average risk, but should be reserved for women with a family history of breast or ovarian cancer, especially if these cancers occurred in family members before age fifty. Test results are not a guarantee that you will or will not develop cancer. Again, this genetic testing is not being advocated by medical experts for women at average risk at this time since the BRCA gene mutation affects so few people, and since the test is difficult to perform and very costly.

Breast Self-Examination (BSE) and Clinical Breast Exams (CBE)

Breast self-exams have not been shown to save lives when they were evaluated in large studies. We know that you are all reading this and saying to yourself, "Are they crazy? Breast self-exams have been taught forever." You're exactly right. We know this study is a real surprise to most of you because of what women have been taught for years. Monthly breast self-examination (BSE) has been advocated by many groups to help reduce the death rate from breast cancer. The theory is that by performing regular, good BSE, a cancer will be detected sooner, and therefore treatment can be more effective, which ultimately results in a lower death rate. Unfortunately, the latest data just does not support this theory. In fact, a few studies, including a major study published in the *Journal of the National Cancer Institute* in 2002, have shown no difference in death rates between groups self-reporting practicing BSE and those who do not. BSE is still a good idea, but it's not going to be a determining factor in whether or not a woman dies. Why? Because by the time a lump becomes large enough for most women to detect it by BSE, it's already been there for quite some time and has had plenty of time to spread.

The present-day practice is to couple BSE with mammography screening. Our advice to women is that younger women perform BSE monthly since they do not get regular mammograms. In this way, if they should detect a lump or change in their breasts, they can see a doctor sooner and increase their chances of surviving.

BSE should not take the place of clinical breast examination by a competent health care provider. The American Cancer Society recommends that a clinical breast exam (CBE) be performed by a health care professional before every screening mammogram. These should take place annually if a woman is forty or older. Between the ages of twenty and thirty-nine, women should have a clinical breast exam every three years. We think this is a good commonsense rule, but it could be done more frequently in women who may be at greater risk.

Frankly, we wonder how often women comply with this recommendation. Are most of them following this rule? We would hope so, but we doubt it. Why do we believe this is so important? Mammograms are not perfect and a skilled examiner can detect lumps of a smaller size than many women doing their own BSEs. Likewise, a skilled health care professional will be teaching the patient the correct way to do a BSE as she is performing the exam and asking key history questions about the woman's breasts to ensure that no important symptoms are overlooked. Getting a clinical breast examination is an important medical practice that we think needs to be high on your priority list.

Mammography

We've all heard the message: Get an annual mammogram, it can save your life. It's a message that doctors and the American Cancer Society have been trying to get every woman age forty and over to hear. Mammography has been around for many years and its value as a screening tool for breast cancer has been debated for the entire time. The conventional wisdom is that if you detect tumors early enough, your doctor can treat them sooner and you'll reduce your chances of dying. But mammography, even at its best, is an imperfect cancer screening test because it does not detect lesions before they are cancerous. We bet this last statement surprises you. Mammography can miss up to 25 percent of tumors in women over age forty. So, why even bother with the test? The big advantage of mammography is that it can detect lesions too small to detect on breast examination, and frankly, it's the best tool that we have at this time that can be applied to all women.

The American Cancer Society advocates that all women at average risk for breast cancer and who are age forty and over have a screening mammogram performed every year along with a clinical breast exam (CBE) performed by a health professional. This is consistent with the new federal government guidelines. The message is definitely getting out, as the percentage of women forty and older undergoing screening has gone from 30 percent in 1987 to 67 percent in 1998. Younger women should undergo CBE at the time of their usual checkups, and if they have further risk factors for breast cancer, they should have mammograms at an earlier age than forty.

There are two kinds of mammography and they are very different.

1. **Screening mammography:** A screening mammogram is an X ray of the breast used to detect breast changes in women who have no signs or symptoms of breast cancer. It usually involves two X rays of each breast. This is the test most women get. If it shows some abnormalities, a diagnostic mammogram will be given.

2. **Diagnostic mammography:** A diagnostic mammogram is an X ray of the breast that is used to diagnose unusual breast changes, such as a lump, pain, thickening, nipple discharge, or a change in size or shape. It is also used to evaluate changes detected on screening mammograms. It takes longer than a screening exam and can focus on specific areas of concern in the breast.

In almost all studies, mammography screening has been shown to achieve the greatest reduction in death rates in women age fifty and older. A recent Swedish study of almost 250,000 women that followed its subjects over many years found that regular mammograms reduced deaths from breast cancer by 21 percent. Women in the fifty-five to sixty-four-year-old age group reduced their risk the most. A reduction in death rates overall of one in five women is excellent and clearly supports the value of mammography in the early detection of disease. What does this data mean for you? It's pretty clear to us. Regular mammograms can reduce your chances of dying from breast cancer.

Here is some more data you need to know that might be a bit disconcerting. Mammography is not ideal even when detecting cancers at stage one. Detection at this stage does improve the chances of survival when compared to finding it at later stages. Many oncologists, however, believe that cancer cells have already spread to the lymphatic system or bloodstream by the time a woman is diagnosed even at the earliest stages. But even with these sobering facts, the earlier cancer is found, the better your chances of survival. So even though mammography is not perfect, it's the best that we have at this time.

Dr. Peter Greenwald, director of cancer prevention at the National Cancer Institute, states that unpublished NCI data indicate that late-stage breast cancer has declined and early-stage cancers have increased. This suggests that we are better at detecting cancer at an earlier stage, and this allows for treatments that have a better chance of being effective.

One thing you should be aware of is that high breast density significantly lowers the ability to detect cancers when present. Once you have a mammogram, you will know if you are a woman with dense breasts. If you happen to be one, you should ask your doctor about having your mammograms read more closely, including using new computer technology.

Mammography Is Only as Good as the Doctor Interpreting The Results

The most critical factor in the ability of a mammogram to detect cancer is the radiologist's interpretation. The sensitivity (ability to detect cancer when present) and the specificity (not to see cancer when it's not present) are directly related to the volume of mammograms read by a radiologist. The more mammograms read by a radiologist, the better the chances of detecting cancer when it is present. In one study, low-volume radiologists detected 65 percent of cancers while high-volume ones found almost 76 percent. Which radiologist would you want reading your mammogram?

Studies cited in a 2002 *New York Times* article indicate that four of ten tumors are missed in some clinics. One radiologist, qualified under federal law, may have missed twenty-five cases in a two-year period. A California physician referred to in the same article was found to be severely inept in interpreting mammograms even after significant remedial training, but continues to work today because there is no law to stop him. It's clearly a failure of the medical system. Dr. Robert Smith, the head of screening for the American Cancer Society, was quoted as saying, "In some settings, mammography is lousy. In others, it's extraordinarily good. There is no reason to do this without doing it as good as you possibly can."

Doctor competency was originally a concern of federal regulators, but a strong doctor lobby kept oversight of physicians in their own hands rather than in the federal government. The *New York Times* article highlighted the failure of physicians to police themselves and to protect many women. Failure to diagnose breast cancer when it was present is the most common cause of medical malpractice litigation today. In one report, half of the cases resulting in payment to the claimant had "negative" mammograms as the underlying reason for the suit.

Here's our advice to you: We'd treat this just like we would when we are being referred to another doctor for surgery. Who would our doctor go to or who would he send his family member's mammograms to for interpretation? Ask your doctor to check into the skill of, and the amount of films read by, the radiologist he or she is sending you to. After all, it's your life we're talking about here.

Besides making sure you get your mammogram read by a radiologist skilled in its interpretation, the most important thing you can do to reduce the chances of a cancer being missed is to have your mammogram reread by another radiologist. This is called a "double read" and improves detection rates by around 15 percent. It's just like getting a second opinion in other areas of medicine. Having a second pair of eyes looking at your films never hurts, and we advise you to insist on it when your mammogram is being read.

Also, numerous studies have shown great variability in physicians' skills in interpreting mammograms. On average, even radiologists who read a lot of mammograms detected cancers that were present only about 75 percent of the time. This means that about one-quarter of all cancers that are present go undetected at the time mammograms are being read. It's another reason why repeating the test every year or two is so important. One test should never be the final answer. Get repeat mammograms annually just in case an early cancer is missed on an initial film.

Computer-Aided Detection (CAD)

Doctors are always looking for something to help increase their ability to detect cancers on mammograms. Computer-aided detection (CAD) of breast cancers using specialized computer software appears to be very promising in this respect. The CAD data shows an almost 20 percent increase in detecting cancers over a single interpretation by a radiologist. The FDA has approved this technology and insurers are now reimbursing for these double readings. This new technology is very expensive, so only a few hundred hospitals have CAD software in place. We predict that in a few years, all mammograms may be reinterpreted or double-read using this technology. After all, what doctor wouldn't appreciate this kind of help after reading mammogram films all day? We know we would.

Controversies in Mammography

About 30 million women receive mammograms each year. National standards were formulated in the early 1990s under the Mammography Quality Standards Act in the hope of ensuring accurate screening mammography examinations. A *New York Times* article in June 2002 found continuing problems: "Far from ensuring high-quality mammography for all . . . the system has promoted mediocre care for all but an elite, or just plain lucky, few." Basically, the Food and Drug Administration (FDA) has failed to do the job they were given.

These federal standards have helped to clean up the industry by focusing on X-ray machines and images. Government-certified clinics are one attempt at ensuring that mammograms will be safe and of high quality. As noted above, the loophole in these standards is the skill level of the physicians who interpret these tests. (Despite this limitation, we would advise getting your mammograms at a facility that is government certified. Just ask them and they will tell you if they are or are not.) Originally, the FDA wanted regular skills tests for physicians and a mechanism to track doctors so as to identify those who did not measure up. These proposals were abandoned thanks to major resistance from doctors. One suggestion that we have is that women need to make it known to their lawmakers that a mechanism for identifying and tracking incompetent physicians is extremely important to them.

Women should know that mammography is an imperfect tool, and even under ideal conditions, one in ten visible tumors may be missed. As we noted earlier, various studies have found far worse statistics. One important thing that women can do is to ask a clinic about the quality-assurance measures it has in place for their mammogram testing program. Do they even have a quality-control program? How is the competency of physician readers assessed? If there are no programs in place, try to find a local clinic that does have one.

Another controversy surrounding screening mammography is the usefulness of these tests. At issue is whether the benefits of detecting tumors early, when they are small and can be easily removed, outweigh the risks, which include false-positive test results and unnecessary surgery to remove tumors that might not be dangerous. Mammography is not perfect, as it misses some cancers and often detects benign lumps. When you look at the data over a ten-year period of screening exams, you see that about 23 percent of women had an abnormal mammogram, of which 80 percent were false alarms. Needless to say, this creates a great deal of anxiety as well as additional testing and biopsies.

Other Breast Cancer Screening Tests

Ultrasonography
Don't waste your time using ultrasound as a screening device. Its primary role should be to help evaluate masses detected by some other means, and it's effectiveness also depends a great deal on the skill of the person who performs it. If your doctor is using this as a screening tool, run—do not walk—to another doctor.

Magnetic Resonance Imaging (MRI)

MRIs are currently used to evaluate palpable breast masses and to discriminate between cancer and scar, but should not be used for routine screening. An MRI that uses a magnetic field to create an image may be useful to physicians in reviewing abnormalities detected in traditional mammograms, and is also useful in women who have dense breasts. The clinical role of MRI should be in evaluating the integrity of silicon breast implants and assessing palpable masses following surgery or when detected by some other means.

New Tests on the Horizon

In spite of its limitations, mammography remains the gold standard for detecting breast cancer. New screening tests that may be even more effective are being developed and may soon be widely used.

The most promising new technologies are:

Ductal Lavage: In this procedure, which is often referred to as a "Pap smear of the breast," a thin catheter is inserted into the mild ducts, the place where most cancers originate, and cells are extracted and screened. Just as with a Pap smear, ductal lavage can detect cellular changes early, before they have a chance to turn cancerous. Most women note that undergoing ductal lavage feels like a slight pinching at best.

It is now an FDA-approved procedure being used in high-risk women and as an adjunct to mammography for those at normal risk who have suspicious lesions on their mammograms. Currently, ductal lavage is not ready to be used broadly. It has many drawbacks—the most significant of which is many false positives. But one day it might become the standard of care for detecting precancerous cells and allowing for preventive treatment just as a Pap smear is now the standard for cervical cancer.

Full-Field Digital Mammography: This process is very similar to traditional mammography for the patient, but electronic detectors are used and digital images are produced that can be easily stored in a computer. The computer then evaluates the mammogram and can sometimes detect lesions that a radiologist may miss. It might prove to be a better diagnostic tool for women who have dense breasts.

Positron Emission Tomography (PET) and Heat Scans: This detection technology can determine whether or not breast cancer has spread by monitoring how the body metabolizes a radioactive sugar substance that your doctor injects into your bloodstream. The reason behind why PET scans seem to work is that cancer cells metabolize sugar faster than normal cells, so they show up sooner on the scan. PET scans are still an experimental tool for cancer detection but may prove to be useful in the future.

Another new technology uses heat technology to detect tumors. All cells produce heat, but cancer cells produce even more. By using what is called computerized thermal imaging (CTI), doctors can separate cancers from normal tissue and more unnecessary biopsies avoided—maybe by as much as 20 percent. Preliminary data indicates an almost perfect ability to detect cancerous lesions using this new technology. Hopefully, the FDA will approve this soon.

RhoC Protein, Cyclin E, and Detecting Metastases

Tumors that spread from the original tumor site to another are called metastases. They can be extremely difficult to detect because they don't cause health problems until they reach a certain size or impinge upon a vital organ. The ability to identify potentially metatastic tumors is essential for defining the best treatment options. Recently, researchers have found two proteins in breast cancers that they hope will enable doctors to tell whether or not a tumor has metastasized.

The first, called the RhoC protein, is found in high levels in fast-growing metastatic tumors, but is rare in normal tissue or slow-growing tumors. If testing for the RhoC protein proves successful in larger trials, women who have slow-growing tumors or benign lumps may be spared aggressive therapy in the future. Wouldn't that be nice?

The other protein that holds a great deal of promise for predicting breast cancer spread is called Cyclin E. Early studies show that it's significantly more accurate than current methods and was almost 100 percent accurate in predicting which women with early-stage tumors would be alive in later years. Testing for Cyclin E protein requires fresh breast tissue, and presently, most laboratories don't have the ability to test for it. Hopefully, more studies will prove this protein's worth for women.

> **WHAT THE BEST DOCTORS WOULD DO ABOUT**
> ## Breast Cancer . . . And You Should Too

1. Learn the risk factors for breast cancer and be more aggressive with screening, especially if there is a history of breast cancer in a first-degree relative (FDR).

2. Maintaining a healthy body weight, eating well, and exercising daily can reduce your risk.

3. Perform monthly breast exams and have yearly clinical breast exams.

4. Have mammography annually beginning at age forty.

5. Make sure that a radiologist who reviews lots of films and has a quality review process in place interprets your mammograms.

6. Ask that a second radiologist read your mammogram, or that it be read by a computer-aided detection system, as this increases detection rates dramatically.

7. Undertake genetic testing to check for the BRCA gene mutations if a first-degree relative has had breast cancer.

Postscript on Breast Cancer

Some recent new research from Europe has shaken many of the previously held theories about breast cancer and may revolutionize the way women who have it are treated in the future. Currently, virtually every breast cancer patient is treated with chemotherapy, hormonal therapy, or radiation because doctors have no way of differentiating those who will be helped by further treatment from those who will not.

Using genetic signatures from tumors, the researchers found that women with good genetic signatures had almost double the survival rate as women who had bad genetic markers. Small tumors often had bad genetic signatures, while large tumors often had good ones. This suggests that some tumors are deadly, and metastasize or spread more quickly even when small. With this new information and more to come soon, it is hoped that doctors will be able to identify subsets of breast cancer patients who will need little or no therapy and others, who will need aggressive therapy even when their tumors are detected early.

Our advice to women: Keep your eyes out for more research on genetic signatures, as it is already changing the way we look at how cancers spread and which ones are deadly.

CERVICAL CANCER

With regular screening, an American woman's lifetime chance of developing cervical cancer is less than 1 percent. Despite this, cervical cancer is the second-most-common malignancy worldwide in women and is expected to kill about five thousand this year in the United States alone. If you take a closer look at all the women in the country who died from cervical cancer, you will find that half of them died because they never had a Pap test and another 10 percent of them hadn't had a Pap test in five years. As physicians, we find it so frustrating and so tragic to see a woman with an advanced case of cervical disease because, with just a little effort, it's such a preventable disease.

Invasive cervical cancer develops in more than thirteen thousand women each year and carcinoma in situ (abnormal cancer cells confined to the surface of the cervix, which have not spread to deeper tissues) has steadily increased to sixty-five thousand cases each year. Most of these cancers could be prevented if women underwent cervical cancer screening.

Studies have shown that the risk of developing invasive cervical cancer is directly related to the frequency of Pap smear screening as well as the duration since the last screening test. **Women who get Pap smears every one to two years are at little risk for developing invasive cervical cancer.** Why is that important to you? Cervical cancer becomes life-threatening only when it spreads and invades the body. Getting regular Pap smears can almost completely eliminate that risk for you.

The level of care that every woman receives must be tailored to her individual level of risk. Physicians will be more diligent and more aggressive with certain tests and treatments if a person has a number of risk factors compared to a woman who has none. Great examples of the latter group are Catholic nuns. They have an almost nonexistent risk of cervical cancer because they possess none of the risk factors associated with it.

Risk Factors for Cervical Cancer

As is the case with other cancers, doctors know that there are specific risk factors that increase a woman's chances of developing cervical cancer. Here are the commonly accepted risk factors for cervical cancer:

- Sexual activity begun at an early age

- Numerous sexual partners (increases the risk of contracting a sexually transmitted disease)

- Oral contraceptive use

- History of a sexually transmitted disease (STD)

- Persistent infection with the human papilloma virus of a specific type

One of the biggest changes in our understanding of cervical cancer came from the discovery of the link between cervical cancer and the human papilloma virus (HPV). Most women do not know that the majority of cervical cancer cases occur in women who have been infected with HPV and have not been treated adequately.

Human Papillomavirus (HPV) and Cervical Cancer Risk

The link is clear: There is a direct relationship between infection with HPV and the risk of developing cervical cancer. Women who have normal Pap test results and no HPV infection have less than a ½ percent chance of developing cervical cancer. HPV infections are much more common in sexually active women under the age of thirty-five (up to 20 percent of sexually active women are believed to be infected with HPV), while cervical cancer is more common in women over thirty-five. This is consistent with what we know about other cancers. It takes a number of years for cancer to develop from the time we put ourselves in contact with a known causative agent. The good news is that women with HPV infections can clear spontaneously through the action of their own immune systems, but only if their immune systems are working properly. If a women is immunocompromised (the immune system is not working properly as a result of disease, AIDS, or medicines they are taking), they are at higher risk for persistent infections, which, in turn, put them at higher risk for cervical disease.

Currently, around a hundred human papillomaviruses are known and about thirty of these have been found around the anus and genital areas of both men and women. They are known to be sexually transmitted viruses. These anogenital HPV types have further been defined as either high-risk or low-risk types based on their association with cervical cancer. It's the high-risk HPV-type infections that seem to persist in women, and it's this persistence that likely induce the cellular changes that then go on to cause cervical cancer. In one study, more than 95 percent of women with cervical cancer had the high-risk HPV virus present. The message to you is you must find out from your doctor what specific type of HPV you have. Seventy percent of cervical tumors are caused by just two strains of HPV—HPV-16 and HPV-18. If you have a high-risk type, you'll be more aggressive in your treatment and the follow-up you need to ensure that your infection has been eradicated. Because there are usually no symptoms in women who have HPV infection, it's important to be tested regularly.

Obviously, your next logical question is: "What are the best tests for finding out whether or not I've got HPV?" Currently, there are several ways: histology—taking a piece of tissue and looking at it under the microscope; cytology—looking at cells under a microscope; and DNA testing—looking at the DNA of HPV by using tissue samples of the cervix. HPV can't be cultured and standard immunologic assay lab tests are inadequate for detection. The FDA has recently approved a test called the HC2 High-Risk HPV DNA test that identifies thirteen of the high-risk HPV types associated with cervical cancer. These new HPV DNA tests are significantly better (90 percent vs. 76 percent than repeat Pap smears in detecting important precancerous and cancerous lesions of the cervix when compared to the gold standard of care—colposcopy and biopsy.

What does this new testing mean for you and why is it important? Let's use a very real example. If a doctor performs a Pap smear on a woman and the results come back abnormal, the doctor is on the horns of a dilemma.

Male Circumcision and a Women's Risk of Cervical Cancer

We're pretty sure that this next little bit of medical trivia will surprise you as much as it did us. Some interesting new research shows that male circumcision is associated with a reduced risk of genital HPV infection in men. Big deal, you say? Here's why you should care: If your male partner has a reduced chance of developing HPV infection, then you will also be less likely to contract HPV. This means that you'll be at a reduced risk for cervical cancer. In simple terms, male sexual partners who are circumcised put women at reduced risk for cervical cancer.

Should she wait a few months and get another Pap test, or should her patient be sent for colposcopy? (See the section on colposcopy below for a description of this most important test.) Now here's where knowing the HPV type should help to make the doctor's decision easier. If it's a high-risk HPV type, the physician would be much more likely to send the patient for colposcopy—the better, more definitive test.

The Pap Smear: A Good but Flawed Test

Dr. George Papanicolaou developed the Papanicolaou or Pap smear test in the 1930's, but it didn't become the standard of care for detecting cervical cancer until the 1960s. Once it came into common use, death rates from cervical cancer dropped by 70 percent. Now the death rate has plateaued and the detection of cervical cancer has changed only slightly. The biggest reason for this detection failure is that women just aren't getting tested. (Please, please, get your Pap smears.) This is not the only problem; there are also many problems with the Pap test itself that women (and some of their doctors) don't know about.

When a women gets a Pap test, the doctor is supposed to collect a representative sample of cervical cells from different areas of the cervix using collection devices such as a wooden or plastic spatula, a small brush, or a cotton swab. (Brushes get better samples than do cotton swabs, so ask your doctor to use a brush when collecting a sample.) These cells are put on a slide, stained, and then looked at under a microscope by someone in a laboratory.

The accuracy of the Pap test depends on the ability of the health care provider to get exfoliated cells from the cervix on the slide. In a variety of studies, the Pap test indicated no disease in between 25 to 50 percent of cases when, in fact, cancer was present. In a large analysis of Pap test data, the Agency for Health Care Policy and Research (AHCPR) and the American College of Obstetrics and Gynecology (ACOG) found that the traditional Pap test fails to detect a significant proportion of cervical disease. There are two major reasons for this: inadequate specimen collection and failure to identify and interpret the specimens correctly. In many cases, the examiner gets only surface cells and fails to get cells that don't shed easily. Unfortunately, there are many other opportunities for error in this whole process of collecting and analyzing Pap smear specimens. Here are some of the reasons why cases of cervical disease can be missed:

■ The doctor doesn't collect the cervical sample properly and/or doesn't get an adequate sample.

■ The doctor fails to collect cells from the correct area of the cervix.

■ The area of the cervix that is sampled isn't the actual area where the precancerous or cancerous cells are located.

■ The slide isn't stained adequately or prepared properly.

■ A lab technician unskilled in interpreting abnormal cells reads the slide.

■ Not enough time is taken to view the slides properly and make a correct interpretation.

Because of these deficiencies, a number of lawsuits have been brought against laboratories and doctors for failing to detect disease in women who had cervical cancer. In recent years, 98 percent of all malpractice lawsuits against laboratories relate to Pap smear results. It's such a problem that the number of lawsuits filed against gynecologists for failing to detect cervical cancer is second only to those filed because of undetected breast cancer.

This kind of litigation has helped to drive the improvements in the way laboratories do business. Computer-assisted programs were developed to reduce the number of technician errors and make interpretation of tests more uniform. The Clinical Laboratory Improvement Amendments (CLIA) of 1988 were drafted to help improve quality within labs and limit workloads for lab technicians.

American Cancer Society's Updated Guidelines for Detecting Cervical Cancer—2002

The American Cancer Society updated its recommended guidelines for cervical cancer screening late in 2002. The ACS suggests that screening begin three years after the onset of vaginal intercourse or no later than twenty-one years of age.

Once cervical cancer screening has begun, it should be performed annually with conventional Pap smear testing or every two years with liquid-based cytology. When women reach thirty years of age and have had three consecutive, technically satisfactory, negative results, they may be screened every two to three years unless they have a history of cervical cancer, have a condition that affects their immune system like HIV, or were exposed to diethylstilbestrol (DES) in utero.

The purpose of screening for cervical cancer is to detect preinvasive cancers before they spread, as well as to detect HPV-associated high-grade lesions before they become cancers.

Liquid-Based Pap Tests

To address some of the problems of traditional Pap smears, a newer sampling method used for analysis of cervical cells, called thin-layer or liquid cytology, has been developed. This preparation method has been shown to provide increased detection of precancerous lesions known as low-grade squamous intraepithelial lesions (LSIL) and high-grade squamous intraepithelial lesions (HSIL). Don't worry about remembering that last part. The FDA allows manufacturers of these tests to claim the ability to detect early and more advanced signs of cervical abnormality better than conventional Pap smear tests. Liquid-based pap testing may be used as an alternative to conventional Pap testing and screening only need to be performed every two years because it's better at detecting precancerous and cancerous lesions. Some of the advantages of the liquid-based technology over conventional Pap smears include fewer artifacts, more adequate specimens, improved cellular sampling and the ability to use the testing material for other tests like the HPV DNA test. Our advice is to ask your doctor to use the newer thin-layer liquid cytology for your Pap smear whenever possible.

Colposcopy (the Gold Standard for Screening for Cervical Disease) vs. Pap Tests

The gold standard or best test for detecting or screening for cervical disease is colposcopy. In this test, a doctor puts a special microscopic device inside the vagina and looks directly at the cervix. The doctor can put a special stain on the cervix to look for abnormal cells and biopsy those that are suspicious looking. Colposcopy should be used as the definitive test for persons with abnormal Pap smears, but not for routine screening.

Colposcopy is used to detect abnormal cells (*dysplasia* is the medical term used to describe these). Dysplastic cells, even though abnormal, are *not* necessarily cancerous but are indicative of potential cervical disease when they are found in cervical samples. A number of studies have shown that the rate of dysplasia or precancerous lesions found in American women using colposcopy is between 10 and 15 percent.

Ideally, if the Pap test is a good test for detecting precancerous cervical disease like severe dysplasia, it should be able to detect most of these problems better than other tests. Sorry, not true. A new study finds that the Pap test detected only half the cases of cervical disease that were identified by using colposcopy and biopsy. Doesn't say much about our reliance on the Pap test for screening for cervical disease, does it? This is one reason why we recommend that women get Pap smears annually. Because cervical disease is slow growing, frequent exams (read annually) will find it even if it's missed the first time around.

Failure to Follow Guidelines for Abnormal Tests and Other Controversies in Pap Testing

If you had a test that wasn't normal, wouldn't you want it repeated very soon to see if your condition was worsening? Well, there's a great deal of controversy in the medical community about this. Data presented at a meeting of the American Society of Clinical Oncology showed that only about 20 percent of women who should have had repeat Pap tests after a previous abnormal Pap test had them done. The evidence indicates that physicians are not following recommended guidelines for treating cervical disease, and as a result, many patients are being undertreated or inappropriately treated. Doctors also can't agree on how to treat Pap test results that show abnormal low-grade lesions or atypical cells of undetermined significance (ASCUS). We'll tell you more about how to follow up on these abnormal tests a bit later.

What is known about ASCUS Pap smear results is that women have about a 10 percent risk of having a high-grade dysplasia (abnormal cells). Follow-up with these results can go any of three ways, but the preferred way is liquid-based Pap smear cytology and HPV DNA testing at the same time. (We recommend both of these tests if you have an ASCUS Pap smear test.) These tests detect more high-grade lesions than a single Pap smear. If either is positive, then go immediately to colposcopy.

Guidelines reflecting the best thinking by medical experts are now available and should help guide physicians and patients to the best possible care. New decision trees are currently being developed that take other risk factors for cancer into consideration, such as multiple sexual partners, early age of sexual activity, and previous infection with the human papillomavirus. (See *www.nci.com* for these guidelines.)

New Vaccines on the Horizon

There's some potentially great news on the horizon for women. Just recently, a vaccine for one type of HPV virus was announced. Because HPV infection accounts for over 90 percent of cervical cancers, this vaccine can have a tremendous impact. There are four types of HPV that account for almost all HPV-related cancers. More vaccines are under development now, but significantly more testing needs to occur before the ultimate benefit of these vaccines can be known and can be applied to the general population.

WHAT DOCTORS KNOW ABOUT
Cervical Cancer . . . And All Women Should Too

---

1. If you have risk factors associated with cervical disease, find a doctor who uses the newer liquid-based Pap smear technique for collecting cervical cytology.

2. Consider augmenting Pap smear testing with HPV testing every two years based on your own particular risk factors.

3. If you do have abnormal Pap smear results, make sure that your physician follows the recommended guidelines for follow-up care.

4. If colposcopy is done, ask that you be checked for HPV infection, and if it's found, tell your doctor that you want it typed to find out if it's a high-risk or low-risk type.

5. If you do have an abnormal Pap test and HPV is present, make sure that your doctor performs a colposcopy exam to look at your cervix.

6. Finally, and most important, get your Pap smears done every one or two years especially as you get older, as it will significantly reduce your risk of developing invasive cervical cancer.

COLORECTAL CANCER

The next cancer that we'll be highlighting is an equal opportunity killer; it's the third leading cause of cancer death in both men and women. Colorectal cancer (CRC) kills more people in the United States and Canada every year than any other cancer except lung cancer. It's the fourth-most-common cancer in the United States. The good news is that it's also one of the most preventable cancers.

An estimated 150,000 cases will be diagnosed this year and fifty-five thousand people will die of the disease. A person at age fifty has about a 5 percent lifetime risk of being diagnosed with it. However, this disease, which includes cancers of the colon (large intestine) and rectum, is both highly preventable and curable if polyps (the most common precursors to this cancer) are detected early.

Risk Factors

Here's some bad news: About 75 percent of all new cases of CRC occur in people with no known predisposing factors for the disease. Unfortunately, this means that people with risk factors account for only 25 percent of all cases. (As you'll see below, it's another reason why screening in general and colonoscopy specifically is so important.) All that being said, here are the risk factors you need to know about:

- Older age
- A positive family history of colorectal cancer
- Hereditary conditions like familial polyposis
- A diet high in saturated fat and low in fiber
- Excessive alcohol use

■ Sedentary lifestyle

■ A personal history of colorectal cancer

Some of these, like older age and a positive family history, you can't do anything about, but most of the others you do have some control over. The key for you: Make some lifestyle changes.

Now here's the relatively good news: Most cancers of the colon and rectum—at least 80 percent—develop from adenomatous polyps. Adenomatous polyps are small growths in the colon that are considered precancerous lesions. They are generally asymptomatic (this is why you undergo screening even without any signs or symptoms). Occasionally, some of them may bleed and you notice bleeding from the rectum. The prevalence of adenomatous polyps increases from 20 to 25 percent at age fifty to about 50 percent by age seventy-five to eighty. The size of the adenomatous polyp is directly related to the probability that it will progress to cancer. The smaller the polyp, the less likely that it is malignant. Fewer than 1 percent of adenomatous polyps of less than one centimeter will develop into cancer, but of those larger than one centimeter, 10 percent will become malignant in ten years, and 25 percent after twenty years. Few adenomatous polyps progress to cancer in one year because change in these polyps is usually very slow and occurs over many years. This is why sigmoidoscopy or colonoscopy is not recommended every year for persons with average risk.

Screening Tests for Colorectal Cancer

Strong evidence exists to support the effectiveness of screening programs for the detection and the prevention of colorectal cancer. Invasive colorectal cancer and its associated high treatment costs may be prevented through detecting and removing adenomas in the colon, as they are generally believed to be the precursors of colorectal cancer. Expert groups (the American Cancer Society, the American Society of Colon and Rectal Surgery, the National Comprehensive Cancer Network, and the American College of Gastroenterology) have developed guidelines for colorectal cancer screening, which they recommend that everyone should undergo, starting at age fifty.

Even though insurance will pay for most of these screening tests, 60 percent of eligible people have not had any kind of CRC screening test. There are a lot of things that discourage people from having it, and embarrassment is right up there at the top of the list. These tests are not easy to use and are somewhat distasteful. People don't like talking about their bowels or stools. Just look at some of the names that we teach our children or are used for fecal material. They're almost like George Carlin's seven dirty words—*poo-poo, doody, poop, caca, BM,* and *number two,* to mention a few. It's time for all of us to become less prudish and more concerned about getting the testing that we need to save our lives.

Another major reason for so many people not getting tested is the major confusion around which screening test to take. There are other factors that explain the low rates of screening: the effectiveness of screening has only recently been proven and accepted by experts; physicians have not been well educated in its uses; and insurance companies have not covered it until fairly recently.

As with other cancers, the earlier a cancer is detected and the smaller it is, the better the cure rate. For instance, in patients with tumors confined to the bowel wall, the cure rate exceeds 90 percent following surgery alone, and no further therapy is needed. Despite this empirical evidence, rates of screening for colorectal cancer are much lower than for cervical, breast, and prostate cancer. They were ridiculously low in one study of people age fifty and older: only 20 percent of groups who should have had fecal occult blood testing and 33 percent of those who should have had sigmoidoscopy. Why are these rates so low? We've already mentioned a few of the reasons, but let's give you a couple more.

Colorectal screening can save lives, but the general public has been slow to push for this type of screening compared to screening for breast, cervical, and prostate cancers. Many physicians' groups have been at the forefront of those pushing for more screening efforts, but physicians as a whole have been found to be lacking when it comes to aggressively recommending CRC screening efforts to their patients. They have dropped the ball in many cases. They're not giving their patients the kind of information they need or they're not aggressively pushing the screening that's needed. It's surprising in one sense because physicians put themselves at considerable risk for malpractice if they fail to suggest screening to their patients, especially if a patient falls into a high-risk category. Our recommendation to you: Don't wait for your doctor. You need to educate yourself about screening tests (that's what we're doing throughout this entire chapter) and then be more aggressive in demanding CRC screening tests. In 2001, the U.S. Preventive Services Task Force (USPSTF) revised its recommendations for screening for colorectal cancer. These and other preventive recommendations of the USPSTF can be found at www.preventiveservices.ahrq.gov.

Because so many people in the United States will develop colorectal cancer at some time in their life, screening for CRC can prevent many potential cancer and cancer deaths. But colorectal cancer screening is costly and requires follow-up for the many false-positive tests that can occur. Colonoscopy remains the gold standard, but your insurance may or may not pay for it. So what are the best tests to screen for CRC? We'll list the most frequently used tests and what they're good for below.

Fecal Occult Blood Testing (FOBT)

In 1993, Dr. Jack Mandel and his colleagues published a study showing that screening with a test for unapparent or "occult" blood in the stool (using a tool called the FOBT or fecal occult blood test), followed by a diagnostic evaluation of patients with positive test results and treatment, could reduce the mortality or death rate for colorectal cancer by one-third.

FOBT is simple and inexpensive and is useful because cancers of the colon and rectum will sometimes bleed, and this test detects that bleeding. The guidelines from panels of national experts suggest that take-home stool testing consist of six tests (two samples of three consecutive stools). It is the rare patient who provides six specimens as a result of the average person's distaste for collecting them. If a single FOBT is done, the chance of detecting a colon cancer if present is only around 40 percent. The more stool tests done, the better the chances. Why? This test will miss many precancerous polyps unless the polyps happen to be bleeding. This is one of the primary reasons why FOBT is recommended annually. One drawback to these tests is that there are a number of false positives, some of which can be caused by food. (Foods that are red in color or contain blood are most likely to affect FOBT. This means beets, foods containing red dye, and red meats.) Your doctor should provide careful instructions on how to minimize these types of problems. Even with these drawbacks, doctors still recommend FOBT as the first step in saving lives from CRC.

Digital Rectal Exam (DRE)

Digital rectal exams are good for detecting lesions and cancers that are in reach of the examining finger. But fewer than 10 percent of colorectal cancers are within reach of a physician's finger. If combined with FOBT, and exams increase the yield of cancer detection, but a single FOBT card will miss 40 percent or more of cancers if present. A DRE should be part of a complete physical examination but should never be a substitute for other CRC screening tests.

Flexible Sigmoidoscopy

Flexible sigmoidoscopy is an examination of the rectum and lower portion of the colon with a flexible, lighted fiber-optic tube. It's been estimated to identify 80 percent of all patients with significant problems. Sigmoidoscopy can be done in your doctor's office, but only after your colon has been prepared and cleaned. Screening with a sigmoidoscope has been found to reduce the risk of death from cancers within its reach by around 60 percent. As a screening test, it is covered by insurance beginning at age fifty and is recommended every five years in persons at normal risk. Depending on your risk factors, your doctor may recommend this test at an earlier age.

Colonoscopy: the Gold Standard for CRC

The National Polyp Study estimated that 76 to 90 percent of colorectal cancers could be prevented by regular colonoscopic surveillance exams.

Colonoscopy provides a visual exam of the entire colon by inserting a fiber-optic scope into the large intestine. A physician specially trained to use a colonoscope performs the exam; he or she is commonly referred to as an endoscopist.

Colonoscopy is the only technique currently available that offers the potential both to find and to remove premalignant lesions throughout the colon and rectum.

(I have a friend whom I pushed to get colonoscopy because he was over age fifty. He kept delaying and delaying but finally got tired of my nagging and got his exam. He had two small cancerous polyps and three benign polyps that were removed. He had no warning signs before this, so he was really surprised . . . and extremely grateful that I'd pushed him. Before this happened, he didn't see the need for colonoscopy, but now he's an advocate for screening and is paying a lot more attention to personal prevention.—Kevin)

Colonoscopy is more valuable than other screening tests for a number of important reasons. FOBT detects only those polyps and cancers that bleed; sigmoidoscopy allows inspection of only the distal or lower half of the bowel; and double-contrast barium enema (DCBE) allows for imaging of the entire large bowel but does not allow for biopsy and polypectomy (removal of polyps).

Colonoscopy requires the colon to be clean, so your doctor will have you use laxatives, oral cathartic agents, or enemas, usually in combination. (Trust us on this, nobody likes using this stuff, but it's the only way to clean out your colon.) Patients used to be awake during the procedure, but now are sedated (most have no memory of the procedure). Transient pain may occur during and after the procedure, but it's mild at best.

As with other techniques and procedures in medicine, competency varies with endoscopists. The ideal exam in colonoscopy is one in which the entire colon is viewed. This is dependent on the skill of the endoscopist and the adequacy of the preparation. Colonoscopy can detect both cancers and polyps, but like barium enema, it is less accurate when the polyps are small. It's estimated to be 90 percent sensitive for large polyps and only 75 percent for polyps at less than one centimeter. Removing these precursors to cancer reduces the numbers of cancers and therefore the death rate from CRC as well.

The downside to this wonderful test is that it's very expensive—up to $1,500—and most insurance companies do not pay for it unless there are clinical symptoms or a family history of disease. If your health benefit plan refuses to pay, speak to your doctor about writing a letter explaining the need. If this doesn't work, and you're over fifty, it's worth paying for yourself.

Computed Tomography (CT) Colography or "Virtual Colonoscopy"

CT colography, or "virtual colonoscopy," provides pictures of the inside of the colon using CT scan technology. It offers many advantages, but there are some major caveats. The advantages are that it's noninvasive and takes only about fifteen minutes to perform. The disadvantages are that it requires the same extensive preparation as colonoscopy, the accuracy of the test is related to the experience of the examiner, and it's more difficult to visualize small and flat polyps. Because of the relative newness of this technology, there have been no studies evaluating its effectiveness in reducing morbidity and mortality of CRC. And if anything shows up on this test, you'll have to have a colonoscopy anyway. We wouldn't recommend CT colography until this test becomes more commonplace and it is shown to have clear advantages over colonoscopy.

So Which CRC Screening Test Would a Doctor Choose?

Physicians used to think that if they didn't find polyps in the lower colon area using a sigmoidoscope, there weren't any problems higher up in the colon. But researchers are now finding that **about half of the people diagnosed with cancer of the upper colon by colonoscopy didn't show any sign of it in the lower colon.** So what are physicians doing? They are being much more aggressive and actively advocating colonoscopy as a screening device for themselves, their families, and their patients age fifty and over. This is what we advise you to do as well. You may have to push your doctor to perform the colonoscopy, but it definitely is the best test for reducing your risk of CRC.

WHAT DOCTORS DO ABOUT
Colon Cancer . . . And You Should Too

---

1. Follow the recommended guidelines for screening for colorectal cancer.

2. Utilize fecal occult blood testing (FOBT) annually.

3. Get a baseline colonoscopy at age fifty unless you are at increased risk for CRC. If so, don't wait. Get one at an earlier age.

4. Make sure that the physician performing your colonoscopy is experienced and is competent in doing the procedure (ask your doctor). The more procedures most physicians do, the better they generally are.

5. Follow the directions for preparing for any screening test, because good preparation means a better examination.

6. "Virtual colonoscopy" can be a very good noninvasive test in the right hands. If you should opt for this test, make sure an experienced physician interprets it.

PROSTATE CANCER

Prostate cancer is the most common malignant cancer in North American men outside of skin cancer. It's second only to lung cancer as the leading cause of cancer death in males in the United States and accounts for 13 percent of all cancer-related deaths in men. There are approximately 190,000 new cases each year and, in 2002, about thirty thousand prostate cancer deaths. The incidence of prostate cancer in black men is 66 percent higher than in white men (234 vs. 144 per 100,000 men) and accounts for almost 20 percent of cancer-related deaths in black men. More than 70 percent of all prostate cancers are diagnosed in men over the age of sixty-five.

Prostate cancer is rarely seen in men younger than fifty years of age and rises rapidly with each decade. Ninety-six percent of all prostate cancers occur in men age fifty-five or older. Men with a family history of prostate cancer are at higher risk than men without that history. Native American men have the lowest risk of prostate cancer. There is no evidence that prostatitis (inflammation or infection of the prostate) or BPH (benign prostatic hypertrophy or enlarged prostate) cause prostate cancer.

At this point, we need to provide a little anatomy lesson to help you better understand why certain tests are done and how they work. The prostate is a small gland about the size of a walnut that sits behind the bladder and in front of the rectum. The prostate gland produces a large portion of the fluid that mixes with sperm to make up the ejaculate.

The prostate gland is made up of four distinct areas or zones. The peripheral zone is closest to the rectum and is the zone where most prostate cancers occur. (This is why physicians perform that ever-so-fun digital rectal exam (DRE) or prostate exam as an essential part of every good physical exam.) "If you never check, than you'll never detect." The transition zone is the next area of the prostate and enlarges when a man develops benign prostatic hypertrophy (BPH). The fibromuscular stroma and the central zone are the other two areas of the prostate. The central zone is where the seminal vesicles are found and where PSA (prostate specific agent; more on this below) is produced.

Prostate Specific Antigen (PSA): To Test or Not to Test

Thousands of men have had their cancers diagnosed with the help of a PSA test. PSA stands for *prostate specific antigen,* a protein produced in the prostate gland and released into the blood. PSA levels in the blood can increase as a result of physical changes in the prostate that can be caused by trauma, infection, inflammation, prostate manipulation, BPH, or cancer. Because PSA is produced by the body and can be used to detect disease, it is sometimes called a biologic marker or tumor marker.

Total PSA has been used as a screening test to detect prostate cancer since 1988 and has proven to be an invaluable, but controversial, tool for clinicians. It allows for early detection of small tumors, but it's not perfect. PSAs don't always detect disease when it's present. There is also debate as to what age to begin PSA tests and what cut off levels are best to avoid false-positive tests and lots of unnecessary biopsies. Newer tests like the percent-free PSA (fPSA) test are now being used to help physicians sort out those patients who are more at risk of prostate cancer when total PSA levels are only slightly elevated or are in the "gray zone" range of between 4.0 and 10.0 nanograms/milliliter (ng/ml). One recent study found that using the percent fPSA would allow for the detection of 96 percent of prostate cancer and eliminate about 27 percent of unnecessary biopsies. We certainly recommend that you ask for the fPSA test if your total PSA exceeds the traditional cutoff level of 4.0.

A simple-to-administer blood test that can help detect cancer might seem like the answer to a prayer, but in reality the PSA test only detects high levels of PSA and that doesn't necessarily always mean cancer. The only way that a physician can tell which men really have cancer is through a surgical biopsy, which is both costly and unpleasant. It's estimated that only one-third of men with high PSA levels end up having cancer. Like other screening tests, the PSA not perfect, but it's the best we've got at this time.

One in five men with prostate cancer does not have an elevated PSA. You can still have prostate cancer with a low PSA reading, and that's why a digital rectal exam is so important (see section below). The PSA is not perfect, so men need to get the testing done annually after age fifty along with a DRE just in case a cancer is big enough to be detected by clinical examination. As with any other disease or clinical problem in medicine, strong clinical judgment on the part of the physician is necessary. The care and treatment of each patient must be individualized.

Screening for Prostate Cancer with PSA and DRE

The American Cancer Society and the American Urological Society have recommended that all men older than fifty be tested annually with a PSA using a cutoff value of 4.0 ng/ml. (See below for a further explanation.) Higher-risk groups such as African-Americans or those with a strong family history should be tested at an earlier age. Both groups support PSA screening in conjunction with DRE (digital rectal exam) since the combination of the two tests is more sensitive for early detection than either test alone. The DRE is the exam in which the doctor inserts a gloved finger into the rectum and feels the prostate to see if there are any masses present (it often feels like he's using three fingers and trying to reach for your tonsils). It's the part of a good physical exam that men look forward to about the same way women must look forward to a pelvic examination.

The cutoff level for PSA testing has been set at 4.0 ng/ml to allow for detection of smaller tumors not detected by the DRE. It is not perfect, as a significant percentage of men with PSA levels lower than the 4.0 ng/ml may have prostate cancer.

Kevin's Comments

One of my good friends had a PSA level that was originally below 4.0. It almost doubled in value but was still below 4.0. His doctor waited six months, repeated the test, and it had elevated slightly again. After another six months, it remained high but was still below 4.0. The doctor finally decided to take a biopsy. He found cancer throughout my friend's prostate, but luckily, it had not spread outside the prostate. My friend has since had surgery and is doing well.

This example illustrates the fact that cutoff levels aren't exact. The most important point as far as we're concerned is that if your PSA levels increase dramatically, even if they remain below 4.0, you need to be aggressive and get a workup done by a good urologist. Initially, this may mean an ultrasound exam of your prostate and possibly a biopsy. We've seen too many similar cases that turn out to be cancer even though the PSA levels didn't exceed the normal cutoff point.

Several scientists have recommended that cutoff levels be reduced so that more cancers are detected. The problem with this is that they will result in more unnecessary biopsies and other tests. Currently, when PSA levels are between 4.0 and 10.0 and the DRE is negative, almost 75 percent of men tested by biopsy of the prostate are negative for cancer. This has been called a diagnostic gray zone by many clinicians. If the cutoff level is reduced, the percentage of unneeded tests will be even higher.

The use of the PSA in screening for prostate cancer, along with improved methods of disease treatment, have resulted in a significant decrease in deaths from the disease. The biggest reason for this is that the PSA allows doctors to detect prostate cancer earlier, before it spreads to other parts of the body. The prognosis with prostate cancer is directly related to the stage of the disease at the time of diagnosis. The smaller the tumor and the more it is contained within the prostate, the better the diagnosis. Small tumors may go undetected by DRE because they are just too little, no matter how skilled the examining physician. The addition of the PSA test to physicians' armamentarium has allowed them to detect these smaller cancers and reduce the death rate.

PSA Levels and Response to Treatment

Okay, you've had your blood test and your total PSA level comes back elevated. What should you do? Fortunately, you don't have to think much about this. You need to get a biopsy of your prostate (your doctor will take a piece of your prostate). The American Urologic Association has made specific recommendations for the use of bone scans, CT scans, and MRI tests based on pretreatment PSA levels. FPSA blood test levels have also been shown to help with determining the stage of the cancer, should the biopsy come back positive.

Another important point that you need to know concerns PSA levels following treatment: Persistent elevation of PSA levels or increases in PSA after treatment have been found to indicate persistent or recurrent prostate cancer. Not a good sign, but at least you'll know that you've got further problems and that your doctor needs to find out where the remaining cancer is.

PSA Tests: Controversy over Diagnosis

A 2002 study published in the *Journal of the National Cancer Institute* highlighted some of the controversy surrounding the use of the PSA test. Prior to its use, many men (36 percent of white men and 28 percent of black men) were shown to have autopsy-proven but nonclinically detectable prostate cancer. Men had cancer but they didn't know it and it wasn't causing them problems, so they did nothing about it. With the advent of mass PSA screening, the researchers used National Cancer Institute records and found that 15 percent of cancers in white men and 37 percent in black men who had undergone PSA testing were overdiagnosed—that is to say, they found cancers that would have gone undetected in that person's normal lifetime since they were so slow growing or so small. So what's the big deal?

The big deal is that the treatment of prostate cancer, whether by radiation or surgery, is not without potential serious side effects, which leave some men impotent, incontinent, or both. Physicians need to help men evaluate the risk of disease versus the risks associated with unneeded treatment, based on the latest medical information. The key issue is whether or not a man is more likely to die of some other disease before the prostate cancer develops into a problem. This is especially important since 70 percent of all prostate cancers are diagnosed in men over the age of sixty-five who have other underlying diseases—coronary artery disease, diabetes, neurologic diseases, or other cancers. No one advocates prostate cancer surgery in a man in his eighties for this very reason. One of our friends' fathers was eighty-four and in great health. Prostate cancer was discovered and his doctor decided not to operate, as it would cause him more problems than the cancer would likely do in the time he had remaining.

> ## WHAT DOCTORS KNOW ABOUT
> ## Prostrate Cancer . . . And Men Should Too

1. Depending on your risk factors, men should follow the American Cancer Society guidelines and get regular DRE and PSA beginning at age 50.

2. If your PSA level tests high, get retested before having a biopsy.

3. If you are taking any drugs (like Proscar) or an herbal product like saw palmetto, make sure to tell your physician before the PSA test is taken, as the results may be affected.

4. If significant changes are seen in a person's PSA level (even if in the normal range), vigorous follow-up should occur; this should include fPSA and a biopsy (taking pieces of the prostate gland) using ultrasound to guide the doctor.

5. If prostate cancer is found, make sure to get an fPSA level, as it will help to guide your treatment.

THE DOCTOR HAS FOUND CANCER . . . WHERE SHOULD YOU GO FOR HELP

Nothing frightens us more than hearing those three little words; "You have cancer." They immediately induce an ice-cold, water-in-the-face shock. Fear quickly grips our entire being. Denial quickly crosses our minds. "It can't be happening to me. I'm too young and I watch out for myself. Maybe they got the results mixed up." We go numb and can't hear anything that the doctor says. Hours, or maybe days later the truth sets in and we know that we need to face reality. We need help in battling this potential killer. Now the question becomes: "Where do I go to get the best help, and to make sure that I get the best possible care?"

Cancer treatment and specific cancer therapies are outside the scope of this book because they change constantly and therapy varies so much from person to person and from cancer to cancer. Treatment must be individualized. This is why we believe you have to see an expert in cancer treatment—a doctor known as a medical oncologist. We also believe that because therapies are changing so rapidly, it is impossible for doctors to keep up with all the new clinical trials or ways of treating cancer. This is why we have provided you the best and most important Web sites related to cancer. You have to do some digging. You have to be your own best advocate.

The first thing to do is to find a doctor who specializes in caring for cancer patients. Here are the kinds of board-certified doctors you want to be referred to by your primary care doctor:

- **Medical Oncologists** are subspecialists of internal medicine who are especially trained to treat all types of benign (noncancerous) and malignant (cancerous) tumors.

- **Radiation Oncologists** are subspecialists of radiology who use radiation to help treat cancer.

- **Surgeons** treat cancer by using surgical operations to remove the tumor (and in some cases the surrounding tissue and lymph system).

All of the above specialists may be needed to treat your particular cancer. The key is getting to the oncologist or specialist to provide the best plan for you and your unique situation.

The National Cancer Act of 1971 authorized the establishment of new cancer centers for basic, clinical, and cancer control research. Today, the National Cancer Institute (NCI) has established fifty NCI-designated centers across the U.S. To become a **Comprehensive Cancer Center,** an institution must pass rigorous peer review and must have a complete range of cancer-related programs—basic research, clinical care, prevention and control research, community outreach, and education. A **Clinical Cancer Center** must conduct programs in clinical research and laboratory research.

Doctors know that these centers promote interdisciplinary care that helps create the newest and most innovative approaches to cancer care. (A list of these NCI-designated institutions can be found on the NCI Web site at www.cis.nci.nih.gov.) Finding a clinical cancer center in your area can ensure the best possible review of your particular case.

INFORMATION SOURCES

www.cancer.gov: This is the Web site for the National Cancer Institute; in our opinion, it provides the best source of complete cancer information on the Internet. It contains information from basic facts about cancer to screening and prevention tools, as well as the latest information on treatment regimens and ongoing clinical trials. It provides very detailed study information at both the health care professional level and the patient level (800-422-6237).

www.yourcancerrisk.harvard.edu: The Harvard Center for Cancer Prevention is a research and education center based at the Harvard School of Public Health whose mission is to promote prevention as the primary means for reducing the risk of cancer. It provides all sorts of information for individuals to help change their modifiable risk factors. Your Cancer Risk is a tool that allows each person to identify their overall cancer risk as well as individual risks for specific cancers.

www.cancer.org: This is the American Cancer Society Web site; it provides basic information to educate the public much as the other sites do, but we found that it offered an excellent section on treatment options for various types of cancers, as well as arranging contacts/ stories of cancer survivors. It also had a special section of rumors, myths, and truths around cancer that is fascinating and most educating (800-227-2345).

www.nccn.org: The National Comprehensive Cancer Network publishes guidelines in cancer care and maintains a database of patient outcomes (888-909-6226).

www.cancerhopenetwork.org: The Cancer Hope Network matches cancer patients with other individuals who have been through the same experience to provide support and insights into the disease (877-467-3638).

WHAT DOCTORS KNOW ABOUT
Reducing Risk . . . And You Should Too

As you've learned above, there are a few specific ways to reduce your risk of cancer. Here are several more general things that doctors know can reduce their risk of cancer. Why not try some of them yourself?

1. **Don't use tobacco in any form:** In the United States, about 90 percent of all lung cancers are thought to be caused by cigarette smoking. Lung cancer is the leading cause of death in both men and women. Basically, you are inhaling carcinogens into your lungs. What can be good about this?

    Cigar smokers or those using smokeless tobacco don't get off easy either. They have between four and ten times higher a rate of cancer of the larynx, esophagus, and mouth. If you smoke, you put those around you at risk from secondhand smoke, and this kills about three thousand nonsmokers a year. It always amazes us when we hear smokers tell us how much they love their children but then expose them to secondhand smoke in their cars or at home. Go figure.

2. **Exercise and maintain a healthy weight:** Obesity is thought to be a contributing factor for cancers of the colon, prostate, rectum, uterus

and ovaries. And what's one of the best ways to help keep your weight down? Exercise is the correct answer.

3. **Eat healthy foods:** Obviously, eating in moderation and choosing healthy foods can reduce your risk of obesity, which reduces your risk of cancer. The American Cancer Society recommends that you eat five or more servings of fruits and vegetables each day and try to choose more foods from plant sources rather than from animal sources. By eating more greens and fibers, you can reduce your risk of colon and stomach cancers. High-fat diets may contribute to the risk of cancer of the colon, rectum, and prostate.

4. **Avoid alcohol or use it in moderation:** If you decide to imbibe, do so in moderation. Drink two or fewer alcoholic drinks a day. If you smoke *and* drink, your risk of cancers of the mouth, esophagus, and larynx increase considerably.

5. **Use Sun Protection:** Skin cancer is probably the most common cancer, but most sources don't list it as such because it's usually not reported by doctors, and it's generally not fatal. Skin cancer is one of the most preventable cancers. Most occur on areas of the body not covered with clothing—ears, face, hands, and forearms.

    Things to do to prevent skin cancer: Avoid sun exposure during the peak sun hours of 10 a.m. and 3 p.m.; try covering sun-exposed areas with clothing, broad-brimmed hats, and long sleeves; use lots of sunscreen that has a sun protection factor (SPF) of at least 15; and avoid tanning beds.

Summary

The key to dealing with cancer is to detect it as soon as possible, when treatment is the most successful. That's been our emphasis in this whole chapter. Get going and get screened. It's all up to you.

The Constantly Changing Face of Medicine and Health Care

There are three things that are inevitable: death, taxes, and change. In the last few years, has your life taken some twists and turns that you never could have predicted? Have computers and the Internet changed the way business is now done? Has the world situation changed in the last several years? We don't know anyone who won't answer an overwhelming yes to these questions. Everyone's life is constantly changing in some way as time passes. Whether we like it or not, change is inevitable.

When it comes to the practice of medicine or the practice of dentistry, the one constant, and the one thing that we can count on, is change. The problem in any profession is that unless you keep up with change, you will quickly find yourself behind the times.

Some of the stories we've covered for NBC News highlight the remarkable changes in medicine that we've seen in recent years. These include the controversy over cloning another human being, blood tests that can predict who is at increased risk for heart disease even when a person has no symptoms, heart surgery without having to open the chest wide open, 3-D images of a person's anatomy with specialized CT scans, small cameras that a person swallows to provide doctors an internal view of the large intestines, and new generations of antibiotics and vaccines to help treat and prevent dreaded diseases.

Soon, the handheld body scanners that we saw used by Dr. McCoy to detect disease on *Star Trek* may move from the realm of science fiction to reality. We couldn't have begun to predict many of the changes that we've seen in the field of medicine in the last twenty-five years.

25 Years of Medical Change

Medical Service	1977	2002
Lasers	Experimental eye use only	Extensive use for eye surgery, skin disease, and heart disease
Anticlotting drugs (TPA)	Not used	Used extensively to treat heart attacks and strokes
Antibiotics	First-generation drugs and few choices	Third-generation and many choices
Radiology technology	Standard X rays; no MRI or CAT scans	CT and MRI commonplace; 3-D imaging available
Health Care delivery	Managed Care Rare	Extensive Use of Managed Care

No doubt the state of the art in medicine will change even more in the next twenty-five years. It will be exciting to sit and watch, and to stay current with all the changes.

STAYING CURRENT IN THE CONSTANTLY CHANGING WORLD OF MEDICINE

Just imagine that in 1993 you began using WordPerfect software for word processing jobs at your work place, school, or volunteer organization. Since then, you've never used another computer software program and never attended any classes to update your computer skills. There are now software programs like Microsoft's Windows for Professionals, Microsoft Windows 2000, or Apple's Jaguar program. They provide so many more benefits, ease of use, and fewer problems. Can most of us imagine functioning without one of these programs on a daily basis? We think not.

Now imagine your doctor finishing his or her residency in 1993 and it's now 2003. The science of medicine has changed just as drastically. We have new antibiotics, new surgical procedures, new ways of treating various illnesses, and improved methods of detecting disease. Has your doctor kept up with these trends? Has your doctor updated his or her education?

FUTURE TRENDS IN MEDICINE

As we've seen from earlier in this chapter, the one thing that we can be sure of is that medicine and health care will continue to change in the future. Every day we hear or read about new research that provides tremendous advances in medicine. Here are some more of the changes that the experts bet are coming in our future:

Medicines based on our genetic makeup (pharmacogenomics): We will be tested to determine our ability to metabolize various drugs in the near future. Doctors will then prescribe drugs based on our unique genetic makeup. Pharmaceutical companies will design drugs for very specific subgroups of people based on their genetics.

Improved radiological imaging techniques: CT scans, MRI imaging techniques, and PET scanning will allow improved methods for detecting disease and learning how our bodies work.

Focused cancer therapies: Cancer therapy has improved greatly in the last decade, but many more medicines will be developed that will help health care professionals focus therapies toward each person and to each specific cancer.

Extensive use of evidence-based medicine therapies: Physicians often drive without road maps in treating specific medical problems even when easy-to-follow guides are available. Focused chart reviews will help physicians improve the medical care they provide and help them to continue their medical education. Future licensing will be based on demonstrated skills rather than on a onetime licensing test.

Laser therapy for cardiovascular disease: Currently, lasers are beginning to be used to open up diseased arteries, but the field is in its infancy. Soon, lasers will be used to avoid dangerous open-heart surgeries and prevent problems from progressing in our arteries.

Gene-based therapies utilizing data from the Human Genome Project: Completing the mapping of the human genome was a major milestone in 2002. Now researchers will use this data to develop therapies to replace missing or malfunctioning genes. Who knows what the end result will be?

We know that these few examples don't even begin to scratch the surface of the changes that we will see in the future, but we don't have a crystal ball (and we certainly admit that we wouldn't have anticipated many of the changes that have already taken place in medicine). What we do know is that we will all be affected by whatever changes do take place. We all will need to change with the times. We will need to keep abreast of technology and continue our education about the field of medicine to ensure that we get the kind of care that we all deserve. We need to ask the hard questions of our health care providers that we suggest in this book.

WHAT SHOULD PATIENTS DO TO MANAGE CHANGE?

How would you like to be receiving medical care that was five, ten, or fifteen years old? How would you like to be prescribed older medicines that are not as effective and have more side effects than never ones? We don't think anyone would. Why take the chance of not having the best and the most up-to-date medical care? Doctors wouldn't do it . . . and neither should you.

Here's what we think patients should do to help manage their own care and stay current:

1. **Stay abreast of the latest advances in medical therapy:** Continue to read and to watch television. Educate yourself and keep an open mind. As we urge our kids . . . read, read, read.

2. **Use the Internet:** The Internet can be a wonderful tool that provides unbelievable access to tremendous amounts of medical information. Check out the Web sites that we provide in the book to begin your explorations. Be critical and be sure to double-check your sources of information.

3. **Share the information you discover with your doctor:** Your doctor may not be as up-to-date in certain fields of medicine because no doctor can know everything about every disease. Share what you've found with your doctor. The good ones will read and explore more for themselves and will appreciate your effort to share your information.

Summary

Medical knowledge changes all too quickly. It's estimated that it quadruples every ten years. Medical education is a lifelong process for physicians. No one person can possibly keep up with it all. It's everyone's job to work together. We, as patients, need to become active participants in our own care. We need to educate ourselves, to ask questions, and be open to what others can teach us. How else can we continue to learn and grow for the rest of our lives? After all, isn't this what makes life fun and exciting?

USING THE INTERNET TO TAKE CONTROL OF YOUR HEALTH CARE

A survey by the Voluntary Hospital Association (VHA) found that the most important thing that patients wanted from their doctor was information. Because patients often feel that they don't get what they need from their doctors, they turn to other sources, including friends, family, and the Internet. That is all well and good . . . we should be researching our medical conditions and trying to find as much up-to-date information as possible (unfortunately, as we've said so often, it's almost impossible for even the best doctors to be current on all the medical changes that are taking place constantly). But we should also be cautious about the information we obtain off the Net.

There are a tremendous number of health-related sites on the Internet. Like other types of information, the quality and the credibility of the medical content that is available can vary greatly.

The credibility of Internet medical information is a valid concern. In 1999, the Federal Trace Commission launched an initiative they named Operation Cure-All to educate Internets users how recognize health fraud. Officials from the FTC believe that hundreds of Internet sites shut down after the agency went after them, demanding that they remove unsubstantiated claims from their sites. The Food and Drug Administration has also significantly accelerated its efforts to shut down fraudulent medical sites. Unfortunately, there aren't enough governmental employees on the planet to adequately police all of the Internet charlatans. One of the main reasons they are so difficult to hunt down and catch is because many of them operate abroad, beyond the reach of both the FTC and the FDA.

The best thing that any of us can do is stick with sites that contain medical information prepared by reputable medical experts who publish in peer-reviewed journals and who have widely recognized health care credentials. Oftentimes, the better sites will have references to articles, books or journals that provide more in-depth information.

But beware: some of the fraudulent sites look very official. It's sometimes even difficult for doctors to tell which sites are reputable and which ones aren't. In an effort to look more like a part of the medical mainstream, many of the questionable sites imitate medical logos and often include the names of well-known organizations to imply direct affiliation with them.

An organization called Health on the Net Foundation (www.hon.ch) has established a set of standards that can help consumers find Internet sites with medical integrity. The Health on the Net Foundation (HON), created in 1995, is a nonprofit international organization whose mission is to guide consumers, as well as medical practitioners, to useful and reliable online medical and health information. For more information, click on the HON-code link at the site.

The bottom line is that you need to be especially careful when relying on information from the Internet. Like a good reporter writing a story, you must consider the source. That's why it's important to know who supports the site . . . i.e., who provides the information. Anyone who has access to the Internet can support a site. That means everyone from the government, medical associations and hospitals, to drug companies and insurance providers, to support groups, charitable organizations or individuals can set up their own site. And every one of them has an agenda—either hidden or direct. The information contained on these sites can be excellent and extremely useful, or it can be very poor, filled with misperceptions, misunderstandings, erroneous facts, or even angry diatribes against some part of the health care establishment that may or may not have a basis in reality.

Getting the wrong medical information can do irreparable harm to the patient, interfere with the doctor-patient relationship, and ultimately may result in poor medical care. To untangle the mess of health care information sites on the Web, here are of our tips for getting the most from your Internet research:

- We think that the smartest approach to seeking medical information on the Internet is to look to university-affiliated sites and well-established medical Web sites like the American Cancer Society (www.cancer.org), the Mayo Clinic (www.mayoclinic.com), Medlineplus (www.nlm.nih.gov/medlineplus), the National Institutes of Health (www.health.nih.gov) and national medical specialty organizations.

- Look to special-interest medical problem groups for legitimate information, e.g., those with Parkinson's disease can help others with the same problem and provide very specialized knowledge from people who have experienced the disease and its associated problems.

- The very same rules that apply to a safe e-commerce site apply to a legitimate, credible medical Internet site: Always look for a Webmaster link and full contact information, including the name of the organization, a physical mailing address, and a phone number.

- Validate whatever information you get from peripheral sites from another source, just to be as safe as possible. Reporters verify their sources and so should you.

- Ask others with a similar medical problem which Web sites they have found most helpful.

- Explore alternative medicine sources. Traditional medicine does not have all the answers.

- If something looks too good to be true, or too simple, it probably is. Avoid sites that sell amazing cures or solutions to your problem. The risks can be enormous if you get bad health information on-line. Rely only on data that has been reviewed, rated or endorsed by medical professionals or expert groups.

- Use your brain. Review the scientific evidence. Does what you're reading make sense?

Here are some of the best medical sites available to you (see other chapters for more sites):

- American Heart Association (www.aha.com): Heart disease is the number one killer in the U.S., and this is the premier Web site for understanding the disease, how to treat it, and how to prevent problems before they begin.

- WebMD (www.webmd.com): This is an excellent site for basic and in-depth medical data and is often used by medical professionals. It provides easy-to-understand information in a format that is easy to use.

- National Institutes of Health (www.nih.gov): This is a huge site with lots of information that is managed fairly well. There is a health information section that is user-friendly and provides clear, well-written fact sheets about common conditions.

- Merck Manual (www.merckhomeedition.com/home.html): This is also known as the *Merck Manual of Medical Information*. It's been around for years as a trusted desk reference. It has now been published in a text-only edition as well as a newer, interactive version.

Both are informative, but the interactive version has color photos, videos, and many other learning features that are bound to impress.

■ HealthSquare.com (www.healthsquare.com): If you want to learn anything about prescription medicines, this is a great site. It contains the *Physicians Desk Reference Family Guide to Prescription Drugs* and the *PDR Encyclopedia of Medicine.* These are excellent references and the *PDR* is simpler to use without much of the scientific language.

■ Centers for Disease Control and Prevention (CDC) (www.cdc.gov): This is the best site for researching medical information for travel to other countries. It will provide information on immunizations as well as disease outbreaks and some general safety concerns about countries. It's also an excellent site to research infections.

■ Health Care for Dummies.com (www.healthcarefordummies. com): This site is based on the book *Healthcare Online for Dummies,* which was authored by the directors of this site. It provides information on medical Web sites to answer most health-related questions.

■ National Cancer Institute (www.cancer.gov): This Web site is perhaps the best general source of cancer information on the Internet. It contains general, treatment, and prevention information related to cancer topics. It also talks about current clinical trials.

■ The Mayo Clinic (www.mayoclinic.com): The Mayo Clinic is one of America's premier medical institutions and provides valuable information on a wide-range of medical topics.

Here are some of the Web sites that medical journalists use when researching their stories:

- EurekAlert! Science News (www.eurekalert.org): This site is a favorite for reporters. It contains breaking research from medical journals and institutions.

- Science Daily (www.sciencedaily.com): The latest scientific research from news releases submitted by leading universities and other research organizations around the world.

- MDExpress (www.mdexpress.com): This is a medical research and news portal created by doctors.

- Reuters Health (www.reutershealth.com): There is a fee to subscribe to the wire service, but there is a no-fee consumer section on this site.

INDEX

Page numbers in **bold** indicate tables.